HEALTH INSURANCE RESOURCES

A Guide for People with Chronic Disease and Disability

SECOND EDITION

HEALTH INSURANCE RESOURCES

A Guide for People with Chronic Disease and Disability

SECOND EDITION

Dorothy E. Northrop, MSW, ACSW
National Director of Clinical Programs
National Multiple Sclerosis Society
New York, New York

Stephen E. Cooper
Former National Coordinator, Health Insurance Information
National Multiple Sclerosis Society
New York, New York

Kimberly Calder, MPS
Manager, Health Insurance Initiatives
National Multiple Sclerosis Society
New York, New York

New York

Library of Congress Cataloging-in-Publication Data

Northrop, Dorothy E., 1942-
  Health insurance resources : a guide for people with chronic disease and disability / Dorothy E. Northrop, Stephen E. Cooper, Kimberly Calder.–2nd ed.
      p. ; cm.
  Rev. ed. of: Health insurance resource manual. c2003.
  Includes bibliographical references and index.
  ISBN-13: 978-1-932603-34-7 (pbk. : alk. paper)
  ISBN-10: 1-932603-34-4 (pbk. : alk paper)
  1. Chronically ill—United States—Handbooks, manuals, etc. 2. Insurance, Health—United States—Hanbooks, manuals, etc. I. Cooper, Stephen, 1946- . II. Calder, Kimberly. III. Northrop, Dorothy E., 1942- . Health insurance resource manual. IV. Title. [DNLM: 1. Insurance, Health—Unites States—Handbooks. 2. Insurance, Health—United States—Resource Guides. 3. Chronic Disease—United States—Handbooks. 4. Chronic Disease—United States—Resource Guides. 5. Disabled persons—United States—Handbooks. 6. Disabled persons—United States—Resource Guides. 7. Medically Uninsured—United States—Handbooks. 8. Medically Uninsured—United States—Resource Guides. W 49 N877h 2007].
  RA644.6.N67 2007
  368.4'200973—dc22
                                                                          2006026757

Special discounts on bulk quantities of Demos Medical Publishing books are available to corporations, professional associations, pharmaceutical companies, health care organizations, and other qualifying groups. For details, please contact:

Special Sales Department
Demos Medical Publishing
386 Park Avenue South, Suite 301
New York, NY 10016
Phone: 800-532-8663, 212-683-0072
Fax: 212-683-0118
Email: orderdept@demosmedpub.com

Made in the United States of America

06 07 08 09 10   5 4 3 2 1

Dedication

This book is dedicated to Pamela Cavallo, MSW, CSW, now deceased, who, as Director of Clinical Programs at the National Multiple Sclerosis Society, recognized that people with disabilities and preexisting conditions must have understandable and usable health insurance information. It was her vision that the information included in this book would maximize health insurance coverage, promote patient rights, and provide strategies and resources for people with chronic conditions as they negotiate our very complex health insurance system.

Acknowledgments

We extend appreciation to those who gave of their experience and expertise to review this book:

Sharon Finn, CCM, RN, MS

Charles D. Goldman, Esq.

Peter Kennedy, B.S.

Deanna J. Okrent, M.P.A.

Jennifer Ricklefs, MS

Appreciation is also expressed to Deborah Kooperman, member of the Greater Delaware Valley Chapter of the National Multiple Sclerosis Society, for her contribution to the material on Social Security Disability Insurance.

■ Contents

■ Preface

Health insurance is one of society's most pressing issues. The United States is the only industrialized nation in the world that does not provide health insurance for everyone. The uninsured as well as those with inadequate health insurance coverage are increasing at alarming rates. In 1992, 38 million people in this country were without health insurance. Today it is estimated that over 45 million Americans lack health insurance coverage—more than 15 percent of the population. Most of the uninsured are under 65 years of age, as Medicare covers virtually all elderly Americans.

In addition to the uninsured, it is estimated that there are another 16 million people who are underinsured, meaning that they have insurance, but their insurance is inadequate to meet all of their health care needs. This is particularly true of those with chronic diseases disabilities. In an informal survey of people with multiple sclerosis (MS), the most frequently cited unmet needs were

■ Medications
■ Home care
■ Rehabilitation services (physical therapy, occupational therapy)
■ Durable medical equipment
■ Mental health counseling

It is assumed that these same problems apply to those with a range of other chronic disorders.

There are many reasons for this lack of adequate insurance coverage:

■ The escalating cost of health insurance coverage, even among the employed with group plans
■ Refusal by some health insurance companies to sell insurance to people with preexisting illnesses or disabilities
■ Seriously restricted coverage for some people with preexisting illnesses or disabilities

■ The large number of people who are unemployed, self-employed, or employed by small companies that cannot afford to offer health insurance coverage

■ Changes in people's life circumstances, such as divorce, separation, or the death of a working spouse

■ Widespread lack of knowledge about insurance options and lack of understanding about how to make one's way through the health insurance system

■ Gaps and weaknesses in the system

Drastic changes are needed in the U.S. health insurance system. These changes may take years to accomplish, however, as change is usually incremental in nature. In the meantime, we need to make the current system work better. We need to disseminate information about insurance options and increase people's understanding of how to navigate our complex insurance system.

This book contains information about a wide variety of options that can assist individuals who are uninsured or underinsured, or who have questions about insurance and don't know where to look for answers. The first section presents an overview of health insurance plans, Social Security, Medicare, Medicaid, and federal legislation that impacts health insurance coverage. The second section includes directories and resources to assist in researching health insurance options.

This book was developed to assist people with disabilities and chronic health conditions, as well as health care professionals, to understand the health care system and exercise their rights and entitlements within that system. It is important that this information be supplemented and updated with local and state legislation and regulations on an ongoing basis.

Dorothy E. Northrop, MSW, ACSW
Stephen E. Cooper
Kimberly Calder, MPS

1

HEALTH INSURANCE: MANAGED CARE AND INDEMNITY PLANS

■ HISTORICAL OVERVIEW

Not long ago, most people with health coverage went to whatever physician they wanted whenever they wanted, and their insurance company reimbursed them a certain amount of their medical bills. Health care consumers or employers had to pay part of the price plus a hefty deductible. When this type of fee-for-service or indemnity plan became too expensive, managed care seemed to be a good solution because it promised to deliver affordable, quality care if consumers, doctors, and hospitals agreed to certain cost-containing restrictions.

Although managed care was not viewed as a viable health insurance option until the mid-1990s, the concept is not new. In fact, its origins can be traced to the early 1900s. Other forms of health coverage existed some 100 years earlier.

The earliest form of health services in the United States dates to 1798, when Congress established the U.S. Marine Hospital Services for seamen. Compulsory deductions for hospital services were made from the salaries of the sailors.

Many early insurance policies protected against lost income due to accidents. The first accident policy, written by the Franklin Health Assurance Company in 1850, provided that for a premium of 15 cents, the policy would pay the bearer $200 in the case of an injury caused by a railway accident. If the accident caused total disability, the bearer would receive $400.

In 1910 Montgomery Ward and Co. provided a health insurance plan for its employees covering illness and injury. The plan, regarded as the nation's first group health insurance policy, paid weekly benefits equal to one-half the employee's weekly salary, with a minimum benefit of $5 and a maximum of $28.85 per week, if the employee was unable to work due to illness or injury.

By the early 1930s, two approaches to health insurance were emerging. The first used the indemnity model[1] and the second was an elementary managed care model; the earliest health maintenance organization (HMO) originated in 1929 at the request of the Los Angeles Department of Water and Power. However, the growth of health insurance was slow at first, with less than 10 percent of the population covered by some sort of health insurance in 1940. The majority of the plans were indemnity policies.

A major shift in medical coverage occurred just after World War II, when health insurance became an important component of employee benefit packages. As the competition for health insurance became more intense, insurance companies recognized that they could charge different rates for different subgroups within the population. People who were employed were generally healthier than individuals who were unable to work and were therefore offered coverage at lower rates.

By the late 1960s, the cost of delivering health coverage had increased substantially, making it a priority to establish a cheaper yet more effective form of coverage. In 1969 the National Governor's Association proposed a national health insurance plan that would utilize HMOs to provide coverage while containing the rate of inflation of health care costs. The Nixon administration, searching for a model to minimize the role of government in managing health care, also saw HMOs as a way to reverse the practice of paying physicians and hospitals for illness rather than for health. The administration proposed legislation in 1971 that would provide planning and startup funds for HMOs. In 1973 Congress adopted the Health Maintenance Organization Act, designed to stimulate the formation of comprehensive prepaid health care programs.

In 1970 fewer than 2 million people, or less than 1 percent of the population, were enrolled in HMOs. Because the cost of health care escalated dramatically during the next 25 years, and the expense of managed care was considerably less than the cost of indemnity insurance, by 1996 about 60 percent of Americans were enrolled in some sort of managed care health plan (the most common of which were HMOs). Since that time managed care plans have continued to grow in popularity, but HMOs have lost favor to plans with more flexibility, such as preferred provider organization (PPO) plans.

■ WHAT IS A FEE-FOR-SERVICE OR INDEMNITY PLAN?

An indemnity plan provides specific cash reimbursements for covered services, and any medical provider can be used. The insured pays a premium, usually monthly, to purchase the policy and pays charges up to the policy's deductible before insurance payments

---

[1]An indemnity model is traditional health insurance coverage in which physicians, patients, or health institutions send medical bills to the insurance company for payment—the classic "fee-for-service" arrangement.

begin. After the deductible has been met, the insured will share approved medical costs with the insurance company; usually, 70 percent of the usual and customary fee is borne by the company and the balance by the insured. Indemnity plans generally pay costs for prescription medications and tests, as well as for physicians and hospitals. They may not cover some charges for preventive care, such as routine checkups.

There are two types of fee-for-service coverage: basic and major medical. Basic protection pays toward the cost of boarding and care while the insured is in the hospital. It also contributes to the costs of surgery, hospital services, and supplies such as prescribed medicine, as well as some doctor visits. Major medical insurance takes over when the benefits provided in basic coverage end. It covers the expense of lengthy, high-cost illnesses or injuries.

Indemnity plans have become increasingly less common in recent years as the cost containment strategy of managed care has been adopted by both employer plans and public benefit programs. It is primarily only within the Medicare program that the majority of beneficiaries continue enrollment in fee-for-service plans.

■ WHAT IS MANAGED CARE?

Managed care is a system of medical management in which patients, administrators, purchasers, and providers are linked with the common goal of improving health care quality and containing costs. It is a broad term encompassing many types of organizations, payment mechanisms, review processes, and collaborations.

In managed care plans, insurance companies contract with doctors, hospitals, laboratories, and other health-related facilities to meet health care needs. Doctors, hospitals, pharmacies, and other providers of care form a "network" of providers for plan members. This linking of health care coverage with providers is the key to how the insured acquires and obtains care.

■ MANAGED CARE PLANS

Health Maintenance Organizations

The HMO is the oldest form of managed care. It is a prepaid health insurance plan that provides specified services for a fixed premium. In exchange, the insured persons, or members, are entitled to comprehensive care, including screening and preventive services, doctor visits, hospital stays, emergency care, surgery, laboratory tests, X-rays, and therapy. Most HMOs require the insured to pay, at most, a small co-payment when seeing an in-network doctor; charge no deductible; and require the member to pay only a few out-of-pocket expenses as long as the doctor, hospital, or other provider used is part of the HMO network. The following are some of the other features of HMOs:

■ The insured can either choose or be assigned an in-network primary care provider (PCP), who monitors the individual's health and provides most of the medical care. Primary care providers are usually general practice physicians who provide basic, or "primary and preventive," care.

■ The PCP has the responsibility of referring the insured to a specialist or other health care provider when necessary.

■ The gatekeeper model requires that referral to a specialist or other health care provider be made by a PCP.

With the exception of emergency treatment, if the insured obtains care without the PCP's referral, or obtains care from a non-network provider, he or she will be responsible for paying a greater portion of the bill.

Types of HMOs

Staff Model HMO. In this plan, the physicians are salaried employees or partners of the HMO and may also receive bonuses, incentive payments, or a share of the profits. Doctors practicing in many specialty areas staff the organization to ensure the delivery of comprehensive care. Such HMOs may even own their hospital systems, although more typically they contract with hospitals and other in-patient entities in their communities to provide non-physician services. This model affords the greatest control over the practice patterns of physicians and typically offers "one-stop shopping" for outpatients by providing a wide range of services at the HMO facilities.

■ *Advantages:* The plan allows for tight management of services and one-stop shopping.

■ *Disadvantages:* The model may be difficult and expensive to establish, the types of care may be limited, and the network is restricted geographically.

Group Model HMO. In this plan, the HMO contracts with a multispecialty physician group to provide all physician services to the HMO's members. Unlike the staff model, however, the group rather than the HMO employs the physicians. The group practice may work exclusively with the HMO, or it may provide services to non-HMO patients as well. The best-known HMO of this kind is the Kaiser Foundation Health Plan. All physician services for Kaiser members are provided by Permanente Medical Groups under an exclusive contract, while the Kaiser Foundation Health Plan performs the HMO functions of marketing, enrollment, and collection of premiums.

■ *Advantages:* This type of plan allows for tight management of services and maintains lower overhead costs compared with the staff model plan.

■ *Disadvantages:* The model can be difficult and expensive to establish, the types of care may be limited, and the network is restricted geographically.

Network Model HMO. This plan generally contracts with multiple physician groups and may include single- or multispecialty groups. Physicians in the model are often required to undergo utilization reviews and other forms of oversight.

■ *Advantages:* The plan allows for tight management of services and carries lower overhead costs than the staff model plan.

■ *Disadvantages:* The model can be difficult and expensive to establish, and the range of care is restricted.

Individual Practice Association (IPA). This type of plan involves an organization of independent practicing physicians who maintain their own offices and band together for the purpose of negotiating with an HMO. Typically, the HMO pays the IPA a single capitated fee and leaves provider reimbursement to the IPA.[2] In this plan, physicians can provide services to both HMO and non-HMO participants.

■ *Advantages:* The plan allows for very broad participation by community physicians, and it is easier and cheaper to establish compared with the other plan types.

■ *Disadvantages:* Management of physician behavior is limited.

Point-of-Service Plans

Some managed care organizations offer an indemnity-type option known as a point-of-service or POS plan. This plan has a provision offering coverage for the use of nonparticipating providers. This can be especially important to enrollees with medical conditions, who may desire the services of specialists beyond those available through the HMO.

In a POS plan, in order for members to use in-network services at the lowest cost to them, the services must be approved in advance by a primary care physician (unlike a managed care PPO, where the patient can select any type of covered care from any in-network provider). When a member goes out of the network with the POS plan, referral by the PCP means that the HMO will pay all or most of the bill.

Preferred Provider Organizations

A preferred provider organization, or PPO, is the form of managed care closest to an indemnity plan. The insurance company contracts with individual providers and

---

[2]A capitated fee is a specified amount paid to a health provider for a group of specified health services. Amounts are determined by assessing a payment "per covered life" or per member. The payment amount is fixed regardless of the nature of the services delivered.

groups to create a network of health care facilities and medical personnel. Members of a group can choose any physician they wish for medical care, but their co-payments are significantly reduced if they choose a provider in the PPO network. Co-payments are fixed, predetermined amounts paid per visit, regardless of the treatment received. Going outside the network means that the member must pay an annual deductible and co-insurance on higher charges.

Some of the features of a PPO are as follows:

■ More services are available than are provided by an HMO, making the care more costly.

■ A co-payment is required for each visit and is generally higher than the HMO co-payment;

■ An annual deductible is imposed and the total out-of-pocket cost is higher than for an HMO.

■ Prior authorization is required for hospitalization and certain outpatient procedures.

■ MANAGED CARE DEFINITIONS, TERMS, AND FEATURES

Certain definitions, terms, and features are associated with managed care and are used in shaping the parameters of a particular plan:

■ *Gatekeeper or primary care provider.* Access to services in managed care is often controlled by a gatekeeper, typically a primary care provider who is responsible for overseeing and coordinating all aspects of a member's care and treatment. Pre-authorization must generally be obtained from the PCP for member referral to a specialist for surgery or hospitalization. Members of HMOs and some PPOs are required to choose a PCP or else one will be assigned.

■ *Preexisting condition.* A preexisting condition (physical or mental) is one for which medical advice, diagnosis, care, or treatment was recommended or received within the six-month period prior to the enrollment date.

A provision under the Health Insurance Portability and Accountability Act (see Chapter 9) states that group health plans and insurers can apply exclusions for preexisting conditions only to a plan member or dependent who

— Does not enroll during the first period in which the individual is entitled to join,

— Does not enroll during a special enrollment period when there is a change in family status or loss of group coverage under another plan,

- — Has never had health coverage,
- — Has had previous health coverage but for less time than the preexisting condition exclusion period under the plan, or
- — Has been without coverage for more than 63 days.

■ Note that the exclusion period cannot extend for more than 12 months (or 18 months for late enrollees) after the enrollment date.

■ *State modifications to the Health Insurance Portability and Accountability Act (HIPAA).* States must have insurance laws that conform to the federal provisions of HIPAA. However, some flexibility is allowed if state legislation is more generous to the individual. Modifications might include

- — A lookback period of less than six months for determining the applicability of preexisting conditions
- — A shorter period for excluding preexisting conditions from coverage (less than 12 months for regular enrollees and 18 months for late enrollees)
- — Longer periods for lapses in coverage
- — Broader categories in which the preexisting condition limitation cannot be imposed
- — Additional special enrollment periods

■ *Co-insurance and co-pay. Co-insurance* requires the insured to share the cost of medical care. Under an 80/20 co-insurance provision, for instance, the health policy pays 80 percent of eligible medical charges above any deductible. The insured is required to pay the remaining 20 percent.

In the event of a large or catastrophic medical expense, the policy may include a co-insurance cap or *stop-loss limit.* This provision places a limit on the insured's out-of-pocket costs in a given year arising from the operation of the co-insurance clause. The annual cap generally ranges from $2,000 to $5,000, and once it is reached, all eligible expenses will be paid in accordance with the terms of the policy up to the plan's overall limit of coverage.

Under a *co-payment,* or *co-pay,* provision, the insured is usually required to pay a set dollar amount (e.g., $10) each time a particular medical service is used. Such provisions are frequently found in HMO or PPO plans, with a nominal co-payment applied to each office visit and to each prescription drug purchased.

■ *Deductible.* The deductible is the portion of eligible medical expenses that the participant must pay before the plan will make any benefit payments. Generally, the higher the deductible, the lower the premium of the health plan. Most non-HMO medical plans (e.g., indemnity, PPO, and POS plans) have deductibles. Once the insured has paid the deductible, the insurance plan pays the scheduled amount for all future covered expenses.

■ *Open versus closed formulary.* A formulary is a list of drugs approved by a health plan and is presumably based on the most cost-effective method of treatment. Some health plans require physicians to prescribe only those drugs listed in their formularies; others allow more flexibility.

In an *open* formulary, physicians and pharmacies are commonly provided with financial incentives to use specific drugs on the formulary list, but the insured does not incur any financial penalties for using non-formulary drugs.

In *closed* programs, which are most prevalent in managed care plans, non-formulary drugs are not covered at all.

■ *Maximum out-of-pocket.* A maximum out-of-pocket limit is the maximum dollar amount the insured will have to pay for covered medical expenses during a specified period, generally the plan year. For instance, if a plan has an out-of-pocket limit of $1,000, the insured will not pay more than that amount for covered medical expenses. The out-of-pocket limit can be reached by accumulating (1) co-insurance amounts only, or (2) co-insurance and deductibles. In determining how the amount is accumulated, neither method is superior to the other; however, it is clearer and less complex to take the word "maximum" as referring to the maximum number of dollars the insured will pay. The maximum is usually expressed using two numbers, such as $3,000/$6,000. This means that a single insured will face an annual maximum of $3,000, whereas an insured who includes his or her spouse in the plan or who has covered dependents will face a maximum of $6,000 of eligible expenses per year. The family maximum is generally two to three times the single amount.

■ *Open enrollment.* The period of time when eligible subscribers may elect to enroll in, or transfer between, available programs providing health care coverage without penalty is referred to as the open enrollment period. Under such a requirement, a plan must accept all who apply during a specific period each year. To find out more about the open enrollment policy in a particular state, contact either the Department of Insurance or the State Health Insurance Assistance Office. The telephone numbers for each state are listed in the Insurance Directory in Appendix 1.

■ *Prior authorization.* Approval must be secured from an insurance company before an insured can receive a medical treatment, test, or surgical procedure. This means that the insurance company will determine the medical necessity of the treatment prior to authorizing payment.

■ *Premium.* The premium is the amount of money an individual and/or an employer pays, usually monthly, to procure health insurance coverage.

■ *Lifetime maximum.* There is a maximum amount of benefits available to a member during his or her lifetime. All benefits furnished are subject to this maximum unless stated as unlimited.

■ MANAGED CARE VERSUS TRADITIONAL INDEMNITY HEALTH INSURANCE: SIGNIFICANT DIFFERENCES

Choosing a Physician. Those covered under an indemnity policy are given the option of selecting any physician they want to see, whenever they decide it is necessary. In managed care, policyholders are either limited in whom they may see (the situation for an HMO) or are given a strong financial incentive to select only those doctors affiliated with the plan (a PPO).

Consulting a Specialist. Under managed care, the primary care provider usually determines whether a specialist is appropriate, by weighing the cost of the specialist with the need for such care. If the PCP does not refer the insured to a specialist, some plans (i.e., a PPO) allow for self-referral. Generally, in a non-gatekeeper plan, one can self-refer without penalty. In a gatekeeper plan, one cannot self-refer and receive compensation. In a traditional plan, the insured can see any specialist whenever he or she feels it is necessary.

Providers within a network usually negotiate a special rate with the managed care company. Therefore, it is important to remember that if a managed care organization (MCO) pays 100 percent of reasonable and customary fees as long as one remains in the network, and 80 percent of out-of-network costs, the difference may be more than 20 percent, as out-of-network providers can charge whatever fees they choose.

Periodic Checkups. It has been reported that only one-third of indemnity plans pay a percentage of the cost of a checkup. In managed care, since the emphasis is to prevent illness and promote health/wellness, the cost of a checkup by a primary care provider is almost always paid by the plan.

Method of Payment. Traditionally, only indemnity plans required the insured to satisfy an annual deductible in order to qualify for any reimbursement. However, a deductible is now a standard requirement of many plans, including PPOs. In an indemnity plan the insured often is expected to pay the physician's bill up front and later submit a claim to the insurer to be reimbursed for a certain percentage of the amount (usually 70 percent). Under managed care, the insured is charged a co-payment, usually between $5 and $20, and is generally expected to pay it at the provider's office. It is generally the provider's responsibility to file the necessary paperwork.

Physician Quality and Qualifications. A managed care plan assumes some of the responsibility in determining whether a physician is qualified when he or she is invited to join the network. It has been reported that over 80 percent of the doctors participating in managed care are board certified. In an indemnity plan, it is generally the insured who must check the physician's qualifications and credentials and make certain that appropriate care is being administered.

Monitoring Member Satisfaction. Managed care plans frequently solicit the opinions of participants as to the quality of care offered. In a traditional plan, if the insured has a complaint, it is left to him or her to contact the provider directly.

■ MANAGED CARE: ADVANTAGES AND DISADVANTAGES

As health care coverage in our country evolves from an indemnity-based insurance system to one focused increasingly on managed care, questions arise about the advantages and disadvantages of the managed care model.

Advantages

■ Because HMOs and other MCOs seek to "maintain health," they think in terms of prevention rather than incidents of illness or injury. They are more likely to cover routine screenings, vaccines, and preventive care in the belief that such treatment can prevent costly care later.

■ MCOs are able to track patients over time and can provide information to PCPs earlier about patients at risk. This allows them to concentrate on the type of care needed to keep patients healthy with the objective of preventing costly medical procedures in the future.

■ Managed care offers a way of coordinating care through a central administration and common working system designed to reduce fragmentation. A common record system can improve the flow of information about an insured.

■ An effective managed care operation simplifies the process of caring for a client and minimizes billing procedures and out-of-pocket expenses.

■ Managed care offers the opportunity to be more creative in developing ways to meet its service obligations. An example is the utilization of non-physicians to perform tasks normally assigned to physicians.

■ To control costs, MCOs often negotiate fees with doctors, hospitals, and other health care providers. The incentive for the physicians and hospitals is a guaranteed patient pool. The plans then offer patients strong financial incentives—lower out-of-pocket costs—to use the health care providers who are part of the network.

■ MCOs often require health care professionals to coordinate their patients' treatment plans with them to reduce costs. This helps to ensure that the plan delivers the appropriate level of care—neither too much nor too little—something fee-for-service or indemnity plans do not claim to do.

- A number of managed care plans have designed systems to eliminate wasteful and redundant medical tests, which some experts say account for 30 percent of America's health care costs.

- If the MCO is an HMO, it will likely use a PCP in its operation. One of the essential duties of the PCP is to monitor the use of physician specialists. With the restricted use of specialists and the creation of alternative forms of care, money can be saved and costs contained.

Disadvantages

- Many managed care programs require that patients see specialists only upon the referral of the PCP. PCPs may also monitor the specialists, (including in-network), depending on the type of plan. This mandate may be no more than a minor inconvenience to the insured, but it could become a major impediment if the PCP feels pressure to restrict access to specialists.

- The insured's preferred hospital, physicians, pharmacy, or other providers may not be in the network.

- If physicians are judged on the basis of their use of laboratory testing, there will be pressure to avoid testing in marginal situations. Many managed care programs use clinical protocols in establishing norms that are often very restrictive in the ordering of tests.

- When the benefit package includes drug coverage, consumers may find that certain medications are excluded because of their high cost. Individuals may first be prescribed a less expensive drug, or a generic drug, before having a name brand drug authorized. This process is referred to as step therapy or first fail. Research also indicates that if the insured does not complain about the less expensive medication, he or she may not learn about alternative medications.

- Just as fee-for-service coverage offers an incentive to provide too much service, managed care has an incentive to provide too little. In instances where there is no clear-cut course of action on the best method of treatment, care often is based on dollars and cents. In other words, the less costly treatment may be used regardless of whether it is the best in a specific situation.

■ DEFINED-CONTRIBUTION/HIGH-DEDUCTIBLE HEALTH PLANS

There is a current trend on the part of employers facing escalating health insurance costs to offer employees an insurance product called a *defined-contribution* or *high-deductible plan*. These plans shift the responsibility for payment and selection of health care services from the employer to the employee.

There are a variety of approaches to the defined-contribution plan concept. In an extreme form, an employer might terminate its group health plan and provide vouchers for employees to purchase their own coverage. In another model, employees would pay an annual premium, probably lower than under traditional plans, and would then receive an allowance of perhaps a few thousand dollars to spend on their medical expenses for the year, including drugs. Once they have spent that allowance, they would be required to cover all costs up to a determined amount, beyond which the employer would again cover most of the expenses.

The advantage of these plans is that they are consumer directed (which is another name for these plans) and give employees the incentive to spend carefully on their health care and receive the best value for the dollar. The disadvantage is that these plans favor individuals who are healthier and have lower medical expenses. Individuals with chronic medical conditions would almost certainly require health care beyond that available from the initial allowance. There is also a concern that employees might forgo certain preventive care and medical services for purely financial reasons.

The defined-contribution plan is a significant step away from the traditional insurance model that spreads risk across both the healthy and the sick. The traditional system is based on the concept that those members of a group who are ill will be covered by premiums paid by everyone else; the risk is shared. In the defined-contribution plan, those with lower expenses are rewarded while people with chronic medical conditions that are more costly must pay more out-of-pocket for their care.

■ HEALTH SAVINGS ACCOUNTS

Defined-contribution or high-deductible health plans are often coupled with a tax-advantaged savings account that can be used to pay eligible medical expenses. The Medicare Prescription Drug, Improvement and Modernization Act of 2003 approved a form of plan for this purpose called a Health Savings Account (HSA). These HSA accounts, formerly often referred to as medical savings accounts, are tax-sheltered savings accounts earmarked to pay the cost of these health plans' high deductibles.

Thus it is now possible to purchase a health plan with a high annual deductible (at least $1,000 for an individual or $2,000 for a family) and couple it with a tax-advantaged savings account. If such a product is offered as an employer plan, both the employer and the employee can contribute to the savings account. The total annual contribution can be as large as the plan's deductible. HSAs can be rolled over from year to year and are not forfeited when one changes employment.

■ HEALTH INSURANCE POLICY CHECKLIST

In selecting health insurance and making the best use of an insurance policy, it is important to understand its provisions. It must be remembered that the insurance is not only for treatment of the disease or disability that is of primary concern. Unless it is a specialized policy (i.e., catastrophic coverage), the insurance will pertain to all general health needs. It is therefore essential to exercise a great deal of care in the selection process. The following is a suggested list of questions to consider in order to achieve optimal understanding of any health insurance contract:

■ Who is covered (i.e., a "qualified individual") under the policy (employee, spouse, dependents)?

■ Is this a managed care plan? If so, how does it work, and how does one learn about the in-network physicians and providers?

■ Is there a waiting period before a qualified individual is covered? Is there a period of time during which a preexisting condition will not be covered? If so, how long is it?

■ How much is the deductible? Does the deductible apply for each treatment or illness, for each family member, or is it simply an annual amount? Is there a separate deductible for prescription drugs? Mental health benefits? Other?

■ Does the insured pay a certain percentage of costs (co-insurance) after the deductible has been satisfied?

■ Must the insured pay a flat dollar amount (co-payment) for services such as doctor's office visits?

■ Is there a "stop-loss" provision? If yes, what is the maximum out-of-pocket amount for a qualified individual before the stop-loss begins?

■ Is there a maximum amount the policy will pay (a lifetime cap)?

■ What types of services does the policy cover?

■ What is the pharmacy benefit? Are there tiers of drugs that require different co-pays or co-insurance? Are all of an insured's medications included in the formulary?

■ What is not covered by the policy?

■ What are the limits on

   — The amount paid for daily hospital room and board?

   — The amount paid for medicine, tests, or other hospital expenses?

   — The amount paid for specific types of surgery?

   — The amount paid for doctor visits?

   — The maximum number of hospital days?

   — The maximum number of doctor visits during a hospital stay?

■ HEALTH INSURANCE TIPS

■ *Be an educated consumer.* It is essential that consumers learn as much as they can about the types of policies that are available. It is no excuse to dismiss this point by saying that the presence of a preexisting condition greatly limits the choices available. This limitation makes it all the more important to know that, although a preexisting condition may put one at a disadvantage, the quest for adequate and affordable coverage is not a pipe dream and there are choices in coverage if one knows the facts. Consumers must find out for what health coverage they are eligible, whether their state offers high-risk insurance and/or mini-COBRA (see reference later in the chapter), the rules behind HIPAA and COBRA, and the availability of coverage from employers; alumni associations; or business, professional, and fraternal organizations. State departments of insurance, voluntary health or advocacy organizations, and case managers can be valuable resources in accessing and maximizing insurance coverage.

■ *Check agents and companies.* One must make certain that agents and companies of interest are licensed to sell insurance in the state of residence.

■ *Review applications.* It is important to list all preexisting conditions on the applications if requested by the insurer and to ensure that all information is correct. False information or misrepresentation of health conditions in the application is against the law and may result in the denial of benefits or cancellation of the policy. If the insurance agent fills out the application and makes a mistake, the agent must be told to complete another application. If there is a mistake after the application is forwarded to the company, the company must be notified in writing immediately. A blank application should never be signed.

■ *Pay premiums annually.* Money can often be saved by paying the premium one time during the year. Service fees can be avoided and discounts for prepayment may be offered.

■ *Enroll in an employer's group health program if one is available.* The coverage available in a group plan is usually more comprehensive and less costly than what an individual can buy on his or her own. There are also more protections for consumers who are in group plans.

■ *Secure an outline of coverage.* One should request an outline of coverage or Summary Benefit Plan describing what is covered under the policy before purchasing insurance. The outline can be used to compare coverage with other policies being considered.

■ *Review the policy after purchase.* One should read the entire Subscriber Agreement , Member Handbook, or Summary Benefit Plan carefully and review the coverage at least once a year. Handbooks can be secured from an employer's Department of Human Resources or benefits administrator. One needs to read the fine print to make certain that policies meet the family's needs. Never assume that a service, therapy, test, or drug is covered.

■ *Pay by check only.* Purchase of an insurance policy should be done by check, money order, or bank draft made payable to the insurance company, not to the agent or anyone else. One should get a receipt with the insurance company's name, telephone number, and address as a record.

■ *Know about the insurance company.* An insurance company must meet certain qualifications in order to do business in a state. One should check with the state insurance department to make certain that any company being considered is licensed in the insured's state. This piece of advice is for the purchaser's protection. Agents must also be licensed and may be required by the state to carry proof of licensure showing their name and the company they represent. If the agent cannot verify that he or she is licensed, one should not buy from that person. A business card is not a license.

■ POTENTIAL SOURCES OF INSURANCE

Finding health insurance begins with an understanding of the possibilities that are available. Eligibility is usually linked to factors such as employment status, age, residence, occupation, and membership in organizational and alumni groups.

Potential sources of insurance include

■ Employer health insurance coverage.

■ A spouse's insurance plan.

■ A high-risk insurance pool, if one resides in one of the 33 states that offer such insurance. Under a high-risk plan, health insurance becomes available to those who are "hard or impossible" to insure. The drawbacks to this type of insurance are higher cost, limited benefits, and the possible imposition of a waiting period before a policy is issued.

■ Guarantee issue states. Five states require all insurers in the state to sell insurance to all individuals, regardless of medical history or health status. These states are Maine, Massachusetts, New York, New Jersey, and Vermont. In addition, Michigan requires guarantee issue from their Blue Cross/Blue Shield provider.

■ Open enrollment periods. A number of states require all health insurance companies licensed to transact business to allow a resident to purchase a policy during a certain period of the year, regardless of any preexisting condition. Information on a state's open enrollment policy may be obtained by contacting the state's insurance department or its health insurance assistance office.

Telephone numbers for each state are listed in the Insurance Directory (Appendix 1).

■ Group insurance through a professional, fraternal, membership, or political organization. An example of this type of organization is Working Today, a national not-for-profit open to individuals who are self-employed. Health insurance through this plan is currently available to members who reside in downstate New York.

■ A health care cooperative. A cooperative is a voluntary organization open to all persons able to use their services and willing to accept the responsibilities of membership without gender, social, racial, political, or religious discrimination. A cooperative is often associated with an agrarian interest, although the common thread among its members could be an association with a different type of enterprise.

■ Eligibility for Medicare, Medicaid, and/or Medicare supplemental coverage.

■ COBRA. If there is coverage through an employer-sponsored plan and one has been temporarily or permanently laid off, has voluntarily left the position, or has had a reduction in hours of work (disqualifying the individual for coverage), insurance might be extended through the federal Consolidated Omnibus Budget Reconciliation Act of 1985 (COBRA). COBRA applies to companies with 20 or more employees. (See Chapter 10 for a detailed description of COBRA.)

COBRA allows qualified individuals to continue coverage at their own expense for 18 to 36 additional months at the group rate, depending on the COBRA-qualifying event. Moreover, the federal Health Insurance Portability and Accountability Act (HIPAA) extends COBRA benefits to 29 months for those individuals whom the Social Security Administration designates as disabled either before the COBRA event or within the first 60 days of COBRA continuation coverage.

■ Forty states have adopted legislation providing COBRA-like protection to employees excluded from the federal law. A review of these "mini-COBRA" policies can be found in Chapter 11.

2

MEDICARE

In 1965 Congress established the Medicare program as Title XVIII of the Social Security Act. Enacted as one of President Lyndon Johnson's Great Society measures, Medicare originally was to be a federally funded system of health and hospital insurance for U.S. citizens age 65 or older. In 1973 the legislation was expanded to include individuals with disabilities who had been receiving Social Security Disability benefits for a period of 24 months. Special eligibility rules for people with end-stage renal disease and ALS have also been established within the Medicare program. In 2003 a pharmaceutical benefit was added to Medicare.

Forty years after the program began, Medicare now offers eligible individuals various options for accessing their benefits. Many people find that combining their Medicare benefits with employer-based coverage, retiree coverage, or a Medicare Supplemental Plan (Medigap) works best for them. Knowing when and how to take advantage of these options in order to get the best value from the program requires a basic knowledge of Medicare and some careful individualized planning.

■ PARTS A, B, C AND D

Medicare consists of four parts. Part A is hospital insurance, Part B is supplementary medical insurance, Part C is the managed care component, and Part D is the drug benefit.

Medicare Part A

Medicare Part A is automatically provided to people who have been receiving Social Security Disability (SSD) benefits for at least 24 months. However, since individuals must wait five months from the time they become disabled before they are eligible to receive SSD payments, they in effect must wait 29 months before having Medicare coverage; this assumes that application for SSD was made at the onset of the disability. (*Enrollment in Social Security as a retirement benefit for those 65 years and older brings immediate access to Medicare.*)

Part A coverage includes hospital costs for semi-private rooms, meals, nursing services, operating room and recovery, inpatient prescription drugs, inpatient rehabilitation, intensive care, and laboratory tests, as well as limited coverage for medically necessary skilled nursing facility care and home health services.

Most people do not pay a monthly premium for Part A because they have met the quarters-of-employment requirement (which includes self-employed work). If qualifications for premium-free Part A are not met, coverage may be purchased.

Part A does require Medicare beneficiaries to be subject to a deductible for hospital stays per benefit period. (In 2006 the deduction was $952.) A benefit period begins the first day of an inpatient hospital stay and ends when the beneficiary has been out of the hospital or skilled nursing facility for 60 consecutive days.

For each benefit period, a Medicare beneficiary (as of 2006) pays under Part A

- A total of $952 for a hospital stay of 1 to 60 days
- $238 per day for days 61 to 90 of a hospital stay
- $476 per day for days 91 to 150 of a hospital stay
- All costs for each day beyond 150 days

Medicare also provides some coverage for a skilled nursing facility (and home health care when medically necessary). The beneficiary is entitled to a semi-private room and nursing or rehabilitation therapies, and for each benefit period the plan pays

- Nothing for the first 20 days
- Up to $119 per day for days 21 to 100
- All costs beyond day 100

Medicare Part B

Coverage under Medicare Part B is optional and is offered to all beneficiaries when they enroll in Part A. If the beneficiary decides to enroll, he or she is required to pay a premium of $88.50 per month as of 2006; the cost of this premium is usually increased every year.

Because Part B enrollment is voluntary, many people who age into the program do not need to join when they first become Medicare eligible because they are still working and have employer-based coverage, or have coverage from a spouse's employer. However, when an individual is not (or is no longer) covered by another plan, he or she must enroll in Part B during the Initial Enrollment Period to avoid a permanent premium penalty of 10 percent for every month enrollment is delayed. An individual's Initial Enrollment Period lasts for seven months beginning three months prior to his or her 65th birthday.

The rules for coordinating benefits when individuals are enrolled in both Medicare and an employer or retiree plan vary depending on working status, age, and the size of the employer group. Medicare is considered the primary coverage for beneficiaries 65 or more years old who are also covered through their own or their spouse's current employer, as long as there are more than 20 employees. (The reverse is true if the employer group is smaller.) Medicare is always the primary payer for retired individuals who also have employee retiree coverage.

SSD recipients become eligible for Medicare Part B when they become eligible for Part A. Part B covers a variety of medical services and is often referred to as the medical insurance part of Medicare. Title XVIII of the Social Security Act restricts coverage and payment to those services that are medically reasonable and necessary in accordance with accepted medical standards.

Services covered under Part B include

- Physician services
- A one-time routine physical exam for new enrollees (within six months)
- Inpatient and outpatient medical services and supplies
- Physical and speech therapy
- Diagnostic tests
- Ambulance services
- Radiology and pathology services (inpatient and outpatient)
- Up to 35 hours per week of medically necessary home health care
- Blood and urinalysis tests

Part B also pays for durable equipment in various ways. Some equipment must be rented while other equipment is required to be purchased. The Durable Medical Equipment Regional Carrier can provide more specific information. The telephone number for the local carrier may be accessed at http://www.medicare.gov/contacts/home.asp.

The Medicare Part B annual deductible was $124 in 2006. After the deduction has been satisfied, Medicare generally pays 80 percent of the approved amount.

Services Not Covered under Medicare A and B

The following services are not covered by Medicare A and B:

■ Personal convenience items

■ Private-duty nurse

■ Private room, unless medically necessary

■ Routine physical examinations and tests related to exams

■ Routine foot care, including orthopedic shoes

■ Dental services

■ Cosmetic surgery

■ Examinations for prescribing or fitting eyeglasses or hearing aids

■ Eyeglasses or hearing aids

■ Most immunizations

■ Most prescription drugs (see the section "Medicare Part D")

■ Custodial care in a nursing home or at home

■ Most chiropractic care

■ Acupuncture

■ Medical devices not approved by the U.S. Food and Drug Administration

■ Non-emergency services rendered outside the United States (Canada or Mexico may be an exception)

Medicare Part C: The Managed Care Option

Medicare Part C—also called Medicare Advantage—is an alternative to traditional Medicare. It refers to private managed care plans that provide Part A and Part B benefits and, many times, additional benefits as well. These plans may be health maintenance organizations (HMOs), preferred provider organizations (PPOs), a private fee-for-service (FFS) plan, or any other type of health plan authorized by Social Security. Generally these plans operate on a "risk" basis; that is, they receive a fixed payment from Medicare for each beneficiary enrolled in the plan. To remain profitable, they must provide the required health care services for less than the amount they are reimbursed.

Except for emergency and urgently needed treatment, Medicare HMOs require the beneficiary to use only health care providers employed or contracted by the plan. Typically, the beneficiary must select a primary care provider (PCP) who acts as a gatekeeper for all health care services. Both the PCP and the managed care organizations are authorized to limit the plan's scope of services (e.g., the length of a hospital stay or the duration of post-hospital therapy services) or the beneficiary's access to specialists and hospitals.

This cost-saving feature also applies in the case of a Medicare PPO. In a PPO, enrollees can choose any doctor, hospital, or specialist offered within the network. If they go outside the plan, however, they agree to share in the cost of care.

Under Medicare's managed care arrangement, plans are responsible for offering a basic package of medical services, comparable to those covered by parts A and B, through a network of physicians, hospitals, and other medical providers. In addition, most plans choose to provide extra benefits. They often offer coverage for eyeglasses, hearing aids, and other medical services not offered by traditional Medicare. The main advantage for the beneficiary is extended coverage and a single, predictable fixed monthly premium with few out-of-pocket expenses.

In some areas of the country, Medicare Part C also offers a beneficiary the option of being covered under an indemnity plan, referred to as a private FFS plan. The insurer, rather than the Medicare program, decides how much to reimburse for services provided. Features of the plan include the following:

▪ Medicare pays a set amount every month to the private insurance company to cover traditional Medicare benefits.

▪ The beneficiary can go to any doctor or hospital that accepts the plan's payment.

▪ Providers are allowed to bill beyond what the plan pays (up to a limit), and the beneficiary may also be responsible for additional premiums.

(The various types of managed care plans are described in Chapter 1.)

Medicare Advantage PPO Plans

Within Medicare Advantage plans, beneficiaries also have an opportunity to choose a preferred provider organization (PPO) plan for their coverage. Although benefits offered in a particular state may differ from those provided in another state, common features of participating PPOs include

▪ Networks of preferred providers (hospitals, physicians, and other providers) who supply all of the basic Medicare benefits, plus additional benefits such as annual physicals, other preventive services, disease management, and prescription drugs.

▪ Unrestricted access to doctors and hospitals without a referral.

▪ A balance of monthly premiums and some cost sharing amounts paid by the plan enrollees. For in-network services, the cost sharing amounts are lower than those for out-of-network services. In some cases, there are out-of-pocket maximums so when this limit is reached, there is no more cost sharing.

- Fees paid to out-of-network providers are no more than the providers would get in fee-for-service Medicare.

- Premiums vary but are priced between existing HMO premiums and premiums charged by Medigap or Medicare supplemental insurance products.

Medicare Part D

Of the various health care needs not included in traditional Medicare when it was established, the most significant one for most Medicare beneficiaries was (outpatient) prescription drug coverage. In response to concern about this coverage gap, in 2003 Congress enacted legislation called the Medicare Prescription Drug Improvement Act and created Medicare Part D to give beneficiaries access to prescription drug coverage.

The Medicare prescription drug benefit is administered through private health plans approved by Medicare. This means that there is no universal prescription plan administered by the government that is standardized for all Medicare beneficiaries. Instead, the benefit is offered through hundreds of private plans around the country that accept the basic parameters established by Medicare but with flexibility in terms of pricing and formulary structure within that framework.

With Medicare Part D there is considerable cost sharing with enrollees, and plans do not cover all drugs. The program requires that beneficiaries make many informed choices to take full advantage of the benefit. Certain aspects of the program are likely to change over time as the result of congressional action or through regulatory changes made by the Center for Medicare & Medicaid Services, which oversees the program.

Starting in 2006, beneficiaries in Parts A and B who wish to stay in traditional fee-for-service Medicare have the option to purchase a separate prescription drug policy from companies offering plans in their area. Alternatively, beneficiaries eligible for, or already enrolled in, a Medicare managed care plan may choose a Medicare Advantage (i.e., Part C) plan that includes prescription drug coverage. (Most people already enrolled in a Medicare Advantage plan prior to 2006 were automatically enrolled in a new, expanded plan with drug coverage as an additional benefit.)

Deciding to Apply

Like Part B, enrollment in a Part D plan is voluntary and anyone eligible for both Medicare Parts A and B may buy a plan. However, unless one has comparable coverage from another source, there is a penalty for enrolling after the initial period of eligibility Therefore, knowing if and when one may need a prescription drug plan should be the first concern. Some Medicare beneficiaries do not need a Part D plan now because they already have coverage for prescription drugs from another source, such as retiree health benefits. However, if at some time in the future those benefits should change, that would be the time for them to consider a Part D plan.

To make this clearer, insurers and employer health benefit plans are obligated by law to inform their enrollees who are also Medicare beneficiaries whether their current prescription drug coverage is *the same as or better than* the standard for a Medicare drug plan. This notification informs the beneficiary if his or her current prescription benefits are considered *creditable coverage* under the law. The notification should be kept with other important insurance documents.

Beneficiaries who choose to stay in traditional Medicare and want Part D coverage can purchase a "stand-alone" private drug plan (PDP). Those who prefer Medicare managed care can choose among various Medicare Advantage plans that include prescription drug coverage (MA-PD). Either way, all plans covering prescription drugs must be approved by Medicare and must give beneficiaries *at least* the standard amount of coverage.

Standard Medicare D Plans

The standard plan set by Medicare for 2007 breaks down *annual costs to the beneficiary* as follows:

- The monthly premium, which averaged $32 in 2006
- An annual deductible of $265 per year
- After the deductible, 25 percent co-insurance for all *covered* drugs (in the formulary) until cumulative drug costs reach $2,400;
- *All* prescription drug costs beyond the cumulative total of $2,400 through $5,451
- 5 percent of covered drug costs exceeding a cumulative total of $5,451

The gap in coverage for annual drug costs between $2,400 and $5,451 has been referred to as the "donut hole" and is a basic component of the design of most plans. Plan enrollees must continue to pay the monthly premium during this time. The "catastrophic coverage" component begins once an enrollee has incurred more than $5,451 in total drug costs in a calendar year (in other words, a maximum of $3,850 in out-of-pocket costs), at which point the beneficiary pays only 5 percent of future drug costs. The Medicare Part D plan is responsible for keeping track of enrollees' cumulative costs, not the beneficiaries themselves.

Other minimum standards that all plans must meet include coverage of "all or substantially all" drugs within certain categories and a network of pharmacies within every enrollee's geographic area. Otherwise, Part D plans are allowed considerable leeway in tailoring their design as they choose in what is currently a competitive marketplace.

Variations in Medicare Part D Plans

Some plans offer lower monthly premiums but higher co-payments, while a few have no "donut hole" but charge a higher premium. Other variations have significant out-of-pocket cost implications for Medicare beneficiaries, which should be taken into consideration when one is comparing plans. Variations include the specific drugs on a plan's formulary, different co-payment levels or "tiers" for high-cost, non-generic (i.e., brand name) drugs, quantity limits per prescription, and more. Because Part D plan enrollees must fill their prescriptions through pharmacies in the plan's network, consumers should check to make sure there is one nearby before signing up.

Choosing a Plan

The variability of the plans available to beneficiaries considering Part D enrollment requires that they and/or their caregivers examine their needs and options carefully. Medicare has created an online tool called the Plan Finder and other information for consumers through their website, www.medicare.gov, to provide consumers with detailed comparisons of Part D plans in a beneficiary's area. If additional information is needed, support is available through 1-800-MEDICARE, from a counselor with the State Health Insurance Program (SHIP) (available in all states; see Appendix 1), or from the plans themselves.

Low-Income Subsidies or "Extra Help"

Congress incorporated into the legislation funds to help make participation in Part D plans affordable for people of limited means. Eligibility for the low-income subsidies (often referred to by Medicare as "extra help") is based on an individual's annual income and assets, and there are different levels of assistance.

Certain individuals are automatically eligible for the assistance, but anyone may apply for it through the Social Security Administration. Application may be done in person at either a local Social Security or state Medicaid office, online (www.ssa.gov), or over the phone (800-772-1213). The application forms and procedures for the extra help are separate from the process of actually enrolling in a Part D plan, which must be done through the plan itself, or online at www.medicare.gov. Those Medicare beneficiaries who are also enrolled in a state Medicaid plan now get their prescription drugs through the Medicare Part D plan benefit. They will be assigned a plan unless they select one themselves.

Penalties for Late Enrollment

All beneficiaries are provided the opportunity to enroll in a Part D Plan when they become Medicare eligible (Initial Enrollment Period). As with Part B, delaying enrollment will result in a premium penalty if one signs up later. Beneficiaries who delay enrolling or who wish to change plans may do so once a year during the Annual Coordinated Election Period (November 15 to December 31).

It is also important for Medicare beneficiaries to be aware that if they enroll in a Medicare Part D plan, they cannot also have a Medigap policy H, I, or J that includes drug coverage. Drug coverage under these plans is minimal and not considered "creditable coverage" by Medicare.

■ FINANCIAL ASSISTANCE FOR MEDICARE PROGRAM COSTS

States have programs that may pay some or all of Medicare's premiums and may also cover Medicare deductibles and co-insurance for certain people who have Medicare and a low income. To qualify, the beneficiary must have

■ Medicare Part A.

■ No more than $4,000, for a single person, in liquid assets such as bank accounts, stocks, and bonds. A married couple may have up to $6,000 in such assets.

■ A monthly income below a certain limit (refer to the following chart). Once a person or couple qualifies, they will be entitled to participate in the following programs:

Monthly Income Limit	Program Will Pay:	Program Name
$858 (individual) $1,133 (couple) (100% FPL)	Premiums Deductibles Co-insurance	Qualified Medicare Beneficiary (QMB)
$1,025 (individual) $1,355 (couple)	Medicare Part B premiums	Specified Low-Income Beneficiary
$1,151 (individual) $1,522 (couple)	Medicare Part B premiums	Qualifying Individual (QI-1)

For more information about these programs, contact your State Health Insurance Assistance Program or 1-800-MEDICARE.

■ MEDIGAP

Medigap, also known as Medicare Supplemental Insurance, is insurance that supplements the basic coverage provided under Medicare and pays for health care costs that Medicare does not pay—such as deductibles and co-insurance. It is regulated by both federal and state law, and, unlike other types of health insurance, it is designed specifically to supplement Medicare's benefits by filling in some of the gaps in Medicare coverage.

Congress has standardized Medigap into 12 basic plans (A to J) to ease confusion over which policies offer which benefits. This arrangement allows beneficiaries to comparison-shop, since insurance companies can sell only the 12 basic standardized policies, although all Medigap plans are not available in all areas. Premiums vary widely according to the plan selected, beneficiary age, and state of residence.

The basic benefits offered under all plans include

■ Hospital co-insurance
■ Full coverage for 365 additional hospital days
■ Twenty percent co-payment for physician and other Part B services
■ Three pints of blood

Each state must allow the sale of Plan A, and all Medigap insurers must make Plan A available. Each of the other 11 plans includes the basic plan plus a different combination of benefits. Although states are only required to allow the sale only of Plan A, most states offer several other plans, and some offer all 12. The plans are standardized to provide the same benefits regardless of what company offers them. *The only difference between companies is cost.* The most popular Medigap plans are C and F.

Enrollment

If someone is a new Medicare Part B subscriber and is 65 years of age, that person is given a six-month open enrollment period for Medigap policies. This means an insurance company cannot refuse to insure the individual because of a preexisting condition. However, the company may make the beneficiary wait up to six months to file claims for preexisting conditions. A Medigap insurance company is also required by law to renew a Medigap policy as long as the premiums have been paid.

There is no federal law that requires insurance companies to sell Medigap plans to people under age 65. For regulations regarding Medigap policies available in your state, either voluntarily or as required by state law, contact your State Health Insurance Assistance Program.

Medigap Plans

Prior to 2006, a few Medigap policies (H, I, and J) included limited prescription drug coverage, but they no longer do. People who purchased one of these policies prior to 2006 may keep it but will have to also join a Medicare Part D plan if they want drug coverage.

A state's Department of Insurance can provide a list of companies that sell Medigap plans in the state. Beneficiaries can also call the State Health Insurance Assistance Program (listed in Appendix 1) or the National Medicare Hotline (1-800-MEDICARE) for free Medicare help. In addition, the Medicare website, www.medicare.gov, offers comparisons of Medigap plans in one's area.

The following chart, developed by the Medicare Rights Center (www.medicarerights.org), enables easy comparison among the 12 standardized Medigap plans. *Note that the dollar figures listed are for 2006.*

	A	B	C	D	E	F	G	H	I	J	K	L
Hospital co-insurance Co-insurance for days 61–90 ($238) and days 91–150 ($476) in hospital; payment in full for 365 additional lifetime days			■	■	■	■	■	■	■	■	■	■
Part B co-insurance Co-insurance for Part B services, such as doctor's services, laboratory and X-ray services, durable medical equipment, and hospital outpatient services	■	■	■	■	■	■	■	■	■	■	50%*	75%*
First three pints of blood	■	■	■	■	■	■	■	■	■	■	50%*	75%*
Hospital deductible Covers the first $952 of hospital charges for each benefit period	■	■	■	■	■	■	■	■	■	■	50%*	75%*
Skilled nursing facility (SNF) daily co-insurance Covers $119 per day for days 21 to 100 of skilled care in a nursing home per benefit period			■	■	■	■	■	■	■	■	50%*	75%*

	A	B	C	D	E	F	G	H	I	J	K	L
Part B annual deductible Pays the first $124 of covered physician and other Part B services per calendar year			▪			▪				▪		
Part B excess charges benefits 80% or 100% of Part B excess charges (under federal law, the excess limit is 15% more than Medicare's approved charge when provider does not take assignment; under New York state law, the excess limit is 5% for most services)						100%	80%		100%	100%		
Emergency care outside the United States Covers 80% of emergency care during the first two months of a trip after a $250 per calendar year deductible, to a $50,000 lifetime maximum			▪	▪	▪	▪	▪	▪	▪	▪		
At-home recovery benefit Up to $40 each visit for custodial care after an illness, injury, or surgery, to a maximum benefit of $1,600 a year			▪			▪			▪	▪		
Preventive medical care Covers $120 per year for health care screenings ordered by a physician but not covered by					▪					▪		

Medicare, such as a physical examination, cholesterol test, or diabetes screening	■	■	■	■	■		■	■	■	■		■	■
100% co-insurance for Part B covered preventive care services after the Part B deductible has been paid													
Hospice care Co-insurance for respite care and other Part A covered services												50%*	75%*
Outpatient prescription drugs													
***Out-of-pocket maximum** Pays 100% of Part A and Part B co-insurance after annual maximum has been spent												$4,000	$2,000

Medigap plans are standardized, but companies sell the exact same plan for different prices. Shop around.

3

MEDICAID

Title XIX of the Social Security Act is the statutory provision that created Medicaid, a federal/state entitlement program that pays for medical assistance for certain individuals and families with low income and resources. One of its crucial roles is the financing of health and long-term care services for low incomes and people with disabilities. According to the Congressional Budget Office, Medicaid is the single largest source of health care financing—public or private—in the United States. Currently, Medicaid covers approximately 52 million individuals. In 2004 Medicaid spending surpassed education as the largest item in state general-fund budgets (*State of the States*, January, 2006, Academy Health).

Medicaid became law in 1965 as a cooperative venture jointly funded by the federal and state governments (including the District of Columbia and the territories) to assist states in furnishing medical assistance to eligible and needy persons. The services that Medicaid covers in most states, ranging from health services to personal attendant care to prescription drugs, are often critical to the ability of individuals to improve their capacity to function and become self-sufficient. Medicaid is also the primary public payer for nursing home care. Medicaid's eligibility rules and benefits are generally structured to provide coverage for those with high levels of medical need, low income, and limited assets.

■ ELIGIBILITY

Three basic groups are eligible for Medicaid:

■ Children, and parents of dependents, who have low incomes

■ Adults age 65 and older who are receiving cash assistance through the Supplemental Security Income (SSI) program

■ People who are disabled, most of whom are eligible because they are receiving cash assistance through the SSI program

The Medicaid Act also allows states to offer "medically needy" programs. A majority of the states have elected this option, thereby allowing individuals to become eligible for Medicaid by spending down their incomes on necessary medical and remedial expenses, including premiums, deductibles, and co-payments charged by Medicare and other health insurance. Within these federal guidelines, states have considerable flexibility in establishing their own financial eligibility criteria.

Many people carry the misconception that Medicaid provides medical assistance to all poor persons. Even under the broadest provision of the federal statute, Medicaid becomes available to the very poor only if they qualify for one of the groups specified by law.

In general, an individual must be an American citizen or a legal alien, meet state income and resource standards, and fit into a covered eligibility category. A person who is disabled, as defined by the Social Security Act, fits into a covered eligibility category unless he or she is receiving Social Security Disability Insurance. The Social Security Act defines disability as "the inability to engage in any substantial gainful activity by reason of any medically determinable physical or mental impairment(s) which can be expected to result in death or which has lasted or can be expected to last for a continuous period of not less than 12 months."

It is also possible to be eligible for both Medicare and Medicaid, even if one is not disabled. Individuals who meet the criteria for both Medicare and Medicaid are often referred to as "dually eligible." As of the initiation of Medicare Part D in 2006, dually eligible individuals must be enrolled in a Medicare Part D plan to maintain coverage for prescription drugs.

■ SERVICE COVERAGE

Federal guidelines require all states to provide coverage of a broad range of basic services. These include the following:

■ Hospital care (inpatient and outpatient)

■ Nursing home care

■ Physician services

■ Laboratory and X-ray services

■ Family planning services

■ Health center (FQHC) and rural health clinic (RHC) services

■ Nurse practitioner services

States also have the option of covering additional services and receiving federal matching funds for those services, which include the following:

- Prescription drugs
- Personal care and other community-based services for individuals with disabilities
- Dental and vision care for adults
- Diagnostic services
- Clinic services
- Prosthetic devices and hearing aids
- Transportation services
- Rehabilitation and physical therapy services

Within broad federal guidelines and certain limitations, states are given the responsibility of deciding the amount to be spent and the duration of services offered under a Medicaid program, subject to the following restrictions:

- A sufficient level of services must be provided to reasonably fulfill the purpose of the benefits.
- A limitation on a particular program may not have the effect of discriminating among beneficiaries based on medical diagnosis or condition.

Under Sec. 1915 of the Social Security Act, states may also request "waivers" to pay for otherwise uncovered home and community-based services (HCBS) for Medicaid-eligible persons who might otherwise be institutionalized. As long as these services are cost-effective, states have few restrictions on the services that may be covered. Services that may be provided under this program include the following:

- Case management
- Homemaker/home health aide services
- Personal care services
- Adult day health
- Assisted living
- Rehabilitation
- Respite care

States have the flexibility to design each waiver program and select a combination of waiver services that best meets the needs of the population they wish to serve. HCBS waivers are expanding and may be provided statewide or may be limited to specific geographic subdivisions. States may also target specific illnesses, such as children with AIDS.

■ MEDICAID AND MANAGED CARE

States have become increasingly reliant on managed care programs to contain rising Medicaid costs and to improve quality of care. In 1991 only 1 percent of the Medicaid population was enrolled in managed care. By 2003 that figure had risen to over 60 percent, or 20 million beneficiaries. This figure continues to grow. Forty-seven states and the District of Columbia now operate at least one managed care program to provide coverage and coordination of care for their Medicaid population.

Medicaid managed care typically means that a state Medicaid program will contract with a private managed care company or companies to provide health care for Medicaid recipients. Medicaid recipients should no longer be forced to rely on government clinics or the emergency room of a hospital to obtain health care. In theory, when Medicaid recipients are placed in the private system, they become indistinguishable from privately insured patients.

One of Medicaid's crucial roles as a safety net program is the financing of health services for low-income individuals with disabilities. About one of every six persons on Medicaid can be classified as a "younger" person with a disability—that is, a child or an adult under age 65 who qualifies for Medicaid coverage because of a disability. Because people with disabilities are a costly population to serve, state Medicaid programs have encouraged enrollment of younger persons with disabilities into their managed care programs.

The state managed care programs generally fall into one of two classifications: Primary Care Case Management (PCCM) and Managed Care Organization (MCO).

Primary Care Case Management (PCCM)

Primary Care Case Management is a Medicaid care delivery model that lies between traditional fee-for-service and risk-based HMO managed care. It builds on the standard managed care model by matching beneficiaries with a primary care provider (PCP) who coordinates care for the enrollee and who serves as a gatekeeper for specialty and other services. Primary care providers who participate in the PCCM program generally receive a monthly management fee, with services paid on a fee-for-service basis. Unlike capitated managed care, the provider is not at financial risk for the services provided. The advantage of the PCCM program is that beneficiaries with disabilities can benefit from the careful management expected from the PCP. Medicaid beneficiaries consume a sizable share of

Medicaid dollars and are frequent users of health services. Any mechanism that can provide better continuity and coordination of care could improve health care for this population.

The disadvantage of the PCCM program is that it restricts choice by placing access to specialists within the purview of the PCP/gatekeeper. Another problem is that the beneficiary's previous PCP might not be part of the plan's network of providers. This may require Medicaid beneficiaries to see new PCPs unfamiliar with their histories.

Managed Care Organizations (MCO)

Managed care organizations (i.e., HMOs) receive a fixed amount in consideration for making available specified health services to a covered Medicaid beneficiary.

Providing health plans with a lump sum creates incentives to furnish care efficiently and to invest in resources that could prevent costly hospitalizations and emergency room use. This arrangement is intended to promote better disease and disability management, and, because the amount received is fixed, there is incentive to use monies more creatively.

On the downside, capitated plans use a network of medical providers, making it likely that some of a beneficiary's previous providers will not be included in the plan. This may cause individuals to sever their relationship with a provider who is not part of the network, creating considerable discontinuity in treatment.

■ EMPLOYMENT AND MEDICAID

Many individuals with a disability rely on Medicaid coverage that comes with SSI for their health insurance. Given the choice of not working—or working fewer hours and retaining SSI eligibility and Medicaid—versus earning a higher income, becoming SSI ineligible, and losing coverage, most recipients would invariably choose to work fewer hours. To counteract this work disincentive, options have been developed for SSI recipients that provide work incentives and allow recipients to continue their Medicaid eligibility.

Earned Income Exclusion

This program allows a portion of a person's salary to be excluded in figuring the SSI payment amount. There is an automatic $20 disregard for any income. After that, the first $65 of earned income, plus one-half of earned income over $65, is not counted.

For example, suppose Joe Smith earns $553 in earned income.

$ 553	Earned Income
– 85	Disregarded income
$ 468	Divided by 2 = $234 (countable income)
$ 630	SSI benefit (varies by state)
– 234	Income to be deducted
$ 396	Monthly SSI check

Impairment-Related Work Expenses

This incentive allows an SSI recipient to deduct from his or her earnings any disability-related expenses that are necessary to maintaining a job, such as personal care assistance, car modifications, or special transportation costs.

Plan for Achieving Self-Support (PASS)

Under the PASS program, one can save or set aside SSI or other income for an occupational goal, such as education, vocational training, or purchase of adaptive equipment. Plans are reviewed every 12 months.

Section 1619b: Continued Medicaid Eligibility

This incentive allows individuals to keep Medicaid insurance even if their earnings become too high for them to continue receiving SSI benefits. If one needs Medicaid in order to work, Medicaid benefits will continue until the individual's annual income is greater than a state threshold level. In 2004 this threshold level ranged from $23,000 to $49,000, depending on the state of residence. Eligibility regarding allowed assets also varies by state.

■ TICKET TO WORK AND WORK INCENTIVES IMPROVEMENT ACT

The Ticket to Work and Work Incentives Improvement Act allows states to make the following changes to Medicaid:

■ Expand Medicaid availability to individuals between the ages of 16 and 64 who, because of income earned from work, are ineligible to receive SSI.

▪ Extend Medicaid to employed persons with disabilities whose medical conditions have improved but who continue to have a "severe medically determinable impairment," as defined by the federal Health and Human Services regulations.

The decision to make these changes to Medicaid is determined by each state. The status of a state's legislation pursuant to this act can be provided by its Department of Insurance. Persons in states exercising these options, who previously would not have qualified for Medicaid, now

▪ Are permitted to buy into Medicaid coverage by paying premiums and other cost-sharing charges on a sliding-fee scale based on income

▪ Could be required by the state to pay a premium if net income exceeds 250 percent of the federal poverty level

More than 30 states had buy-in programs in 2005. Because there are now a variety of ways in which an individual may qualify for programs such as Medicaid Case Management, Ticket to Work, and others that can help provide access to needed medical services, it is particularly important for people with no health insurance coverage to examine their potential eligibility for any or all of these programs. For additional information and guidance on applying for Medicaid and related Medicaid programs, contact the state Medicaid office (often administered by the Department of Health or Social Welfare or Social Services).

4

SOCIAL SECURITY DISABILITY INSURANCE

Social Security Disability insurance (SSDI) is a program for workers unable to work due to long-term disability. It is administered by the Social Security Administration (SSA) and funded by the Federal Income Contribution Act (FICA) tax, which is withheld from workers' pay, and by employer contributions.

If a person earns enough work "credits," he or she becomes insured for disability benefits. Social Security assigns credits for the amount of earnings that an individual receives and on which he or she pays taxes into the Social Security Trust Fund. Each year the amount of earnings needed to earn one credit changes. A person can earn up to four credits per year.

The number of work credits needed by an individual for disability benefits depends on when the person becomes disabled. Generally, the applicant needs 40 credits, 20 of which must be earned in the last 10 years, ending with the year when the disability occurs. Younger workers may qualify with fewer hours. The rules are as follows:

- *Before age 24:* An applicant may qualify if he or she has six credits earned in the three-year period ending when the disability starts.

- *Age 24 to 31:* An applicant may qualify if he or she has credit for having worked half of the time between age 21 and the outset of the disability. For example, if the individual becomes disabled at age 27, he or she needs credit for three years of work (12 credits) out of the past six years (between ages 21 and 27).

- *Age 31 or older:* In general, the applicant will need to have the number of work credits indicated in the following chart. Normally, to qualify for SSDI, one needs 40 credits during his or her lifetime (10 years), with 20 of those credits (5 years) earned within the last 10 years.

Born after 1929 and Became Disabled at Age:	Credits Needed
31–42	20
44	22
46	24
48	26
50	28
52	30
54	32
56	34
58	36
60	38
62 or older	40

■ APPLICATION

Applicants can receive extensive information on SSDI from the Social Security Administration (SSA) website: www.socialsecurity.gov. The website gives an overview of the application process and all of the steps involved. It also provides the opportunity for an online application if that is preferred.

One can also telephone the SSA and arrange for an appointment to initiate the application process. The toll-free number is 1-800-772-1213. Representatives are available from 7:00 am to 7:00 pm each business day.

An individual should apply for SSDI when he or she has been out of work, or expects to be out of work, because of a disability for 12 continuous months. The SSA considers a person disabled if

■ The individual lacks the ability to engage in any substantial gainful activity.

■ The incapacity is due to one or more medically determinable physical or mental impairments.

■ The incapacity has lasted, or can be expected to last, for a continuous period of at least 12 months or is expected to result in death.

The first step in the application process is called the "initial application." It takes 60 to 90 days to process the paperwork. An applicant may shorten the process by submitting certain documents needed by the SSA to help establish disability:

■ Names, addresses, and phone numbers of doctors, therapists, hospitals, clinics, and institutions that treated the applicant, along with the dates of treatment

■ Names of all medications being taken

- Medical records from doctors, therapists, hospitals, clinics, and caseworkers
- Letters and reports, from at least one doctor, based on a recent examination that
  - Establishes the diagnosis of the illness or injury causing severe interference with work activity
  - Explains how the individual meets the impairment criteria established by the SSA for that diagnosis
  - Verifies that the disability will either result in death or is expected to last for at least 12 months
- Laboratory and test results
- A summary of where the applicant worked or works and the nature of the work
- A copy of the individual's W-2 Form or, if self-employed, his or her federal income tax return for the past year

It is also suggested that the applicant submit at this time a certified copy of his or her birth certificate or other proof of citizenship. As the application process progresses, the candidate may be asked to provide additional information on work history, evidence of military service, proof of military discharge, certified copies of birth certificates of eligible children, workers' compensation award information, or a voided check for direct deposit.

Federal statute provides that the same standard applies in determining disability under both SSDI and SSI. Social Security uses a multistep process in determining disability. This process is primarily focused on diagnosis and on whether a person meets the criteria of listed impairments established by the SSA for that diagnosis. If disability cannot be determined on this basis, determination is based on "Residual Functional Capacity" and what the individual can and cannot do in the workplace.

Questions that need to be answered regarding functioning include the following:

- Does the applicant have a severe impairment?
- Is the applicant not working or expected not to work?
- Is the applicant engaged in any substantial gainful activity?
- Is the applicant capable of performing relevant work?

A benchmark used by the SSA, in the event the applicant is working, is that Social Security does not consider the individual disabled if he or she is working in substantial gainful employment and his or her earnings average more than $860 a month (as of 2006).

It is essential that applicants keep track of their daily activities as part of the application process. They must create a clear mental picture of the problems they face, which in turn must be conveyed to the Social Security representative at the time of application. It is important to convey the symptoms that an individual has on his or her worst day, not the best day, and to be as comprehensive and descriptive as possible. See Chapter 6 for further discussion about preparing for the application process.

■ APPEALS

If an application for SSDI benefits is denied (or, if an earlier approval has had benefits reduced or terminated), the applicant or recipient is entitled to appeal this decision and to seek to have the decision reversed. Although some changes in the appeal process are planned by the SSA in the future, steps of appeal currently include the following:

1. After an initial finding is made that is adverse to the claimant, that individual has 60 days to request reconsideration. The claim is then assigned to an SSA representative who did not participate in the original decision. If the request for reconsideration is made within 10 days of the denial, the claimant's benefits, if already in place, will continue until the reconsideration is made.

2. If reconsideration is unsuccessful, the claimant has the right to request a hearing before an administrative law judge (ALJ). This is similar to a court hearing or trial, but less formal. Testimony is taken under oath, and the parties are permitted to submit evidence.

3. If an adverse decision is rendered, the claimant has the right to request a review by the Social Security Appeals Council in Washington, D.C. This must be done within 60 days after the date of the determination.

4. The Appeals Council may affirm, modify, or reverse the decision of the ALJ, or it may send the case back to the ALJ for further action. Once the council renders a decision, the claimant has the right to obtain further review by filing suit within 60 days in a United States District Court.

According to a ruling on June 5, 2000, by the United States Supreme Court, claimants bringing appeals to the federal district court may raise additional issues that were not brought up during earlier SSA appeals.

There are two reasons an SSDI applicant should appeal an adverse decision rendered at either the initial finding stage or by the ALJ. First, according to the National Organization of Social Security Claimant Representatives (NOSSCR), 40 percent of the initial applications for SSD are denied. Of those that are rejected, 20 percent are successful at reconsideration, and over 50 percent are successful at the disability hearing.

The second reason is due to a policy recently implemented by the SSA. If the individual has been unsuccessful at the initial finding stage, followed by an adverse ruling rendered by an ALJ (Stage 2), the SSA now allows the claimant to file a new

SSDI application. Prior to this change, an applicant had to wait until the Appeals Council ruled on the appeal. According to one commentator, this tribunal generally upheld the ALJ's decision and had a backlog of at least 12 to 15 months between the time the papers were submitted and when a decision was rendered. During this period, the applicant would be ineligible to receive SSDI benefits or have access to Medicare and would be barred from filing a new application.[1]

As an alternative, the applicant could file a new application, but by doing so, he or she would forgo the appeal. This was the recommended course if he/she had a new doctor or attorney, or any new medical evidence that was more persuasive in establishing his or her right to SSDI. However, the problem with starting over was that any rights to benefits that the applicant had prior to the new application were lost.

Under the new policy, a subsequent claim will be processed and adjudicated, even if there is a prior claim pending at the Appeals Council. This makes it possible for the applicant to be able to win benefits under a new claim even before the appeal on the old one is heard.

If the subsequent application is approved, a favorable outcome might sway the Appeals Council to approve those expenses incurred prior to the second claim and set forth in the initial application. Each case is considered separately, and if the Appeals Council decides that the subsequent claim presents new and material evidence relating to the period prior to the date of the ALJ decision, such new evidence may be used in the Appeal Council's review of the prior claim.[2]

The law provides that disability benefits for workers usually cannot begin for five months after the established onset of the disability. If the beneficiary leaves the disability rolls and returns with the same impairment, or a related impairment, within five years, Social Security does not require a new waiting period. A beneficiary may also receive SSDI benefits retroactive to one year from the date the application was filed. The five-month waiting period still applies, however.

Should Counsel Be Retained During the Application Process?

No one likes to pay attorney fees. This is especially true in an application for SSDI benefits when the claimant has been diagnosed with a condition that meets one of Social Security's listed impairments. Learning this, the applicant might assume that the application will be swiftly approved after proof of the diagnosis is submitted to the agency. Unfortunately, however, it is not that simple.

---

[1] *Winning SSDI While You Wait for an Appeal*, About Dot Com, 2000, p. 1, http: //chronicfatigue.about. com/health/chronicfatigue/library/weekly/aa02600a.htm?rnk=r1&terms=SSDI+Appeals.

[2] Id. at p. 2.

The SSA requires that an individual be unable to engage in any substantial gainful activity by reason of a medically determinable physical or medical impairment. The condition must be expected to last for a continuous period of not less than 12 months or result in death. Therefore, determination of benefits is based on impairment and functioning, not on diagnosis alone. The immediate question is whether the claimant has the skill to present the necessary proof of this impairment to Social Security without legal assistance. And, assuming the applicant possesses this requisite expertise, will the claimant be able to exercise sufficient emotional control if his or her integrity is questioned? (For a detailed discussion of these issues, see Perkins and Perkins, *Multiple Sclerosis: Your Legal Rights*, 1999, Demos.)

Another factor is the slow pace set by the SSA in reaching a decision. For instance, it generally takes at least three to five months for Social Security to gather all of the necessary evidence and to conduct a hearing before rendering a decision. A skillful attorney knows the roadblocks characteristic of the initial application process and how to avoid them.

It is fair to say that every case is different and an attorney's role depends on the particular facts of the case. However, some of the things an attorney may do can be very time-consuming to the novice, including the following:

■ Gather medical and other evidence.

■ Analyze the case under Social Security regulations.

■ Refer the client to additional doctors whom the attorney has used previously and whose work he or she trusts.

■ Send the client to a vocational expert for a report on his or her ability to work.

■ Request subpoenas to ensure the presence of crucial witnesses or documents at the hearing.

■ Protect the client's right to a fair hearing by objecting to improper evidence and procedures.

■ Advise the client how best to prepare himself or herself to testify at the hearing.

■ Present a closing statement at the hearing arguing that the client is entitled to benefits under the Social Security regulations.

An attorney is strongly recommended when an appeal is necessary. Whether one should be retained at the beginning of the application process depends on the expertise and ability of the applicant to negotiate this lengthy and cumbersome process. It is essential that, if an attorney is retained, he or she should be knowledgeable of the SSDI application process and have experience representing individuals pursuing SSDI claims. The NOSSCR is one resource for finding such an attorney.

■ ATTORNEY FEES

Social Security has two methods of authorizing attorney fees: the fee agreement and the fee petition process. Both methods are dependent on the claimant's receiving a favorable determination. Thus, no money is required "up front."

The agreement process requires the claimant and attorney to file a written agreement with the SSA before the date on which the SSA makes a decision on the application. The fee is usually approved if it is limited to 25 percent of past-due benefits or $5,300, whichever is less. The fee will be paid only if the SSA renders a favorable determination and the claim results in past-due benefits.

A fee greater than $5,300 can be authorized only in cases in which the attorney appeals the fee award and files a fee petition. The amount of the fee authorized under the fee petition process is based on several factors, including but not limited to the following:

- The complexity of the case
- The extent and type of services that the attorney performed
- The amount of time spent by the attorney

■ WAITING PERIOD

Successful claimants for SSDI are subject to a five-month waiting period prior to receipt of disability benefits. Therefore, if a claimant has been awarded benefits with an onset date of February 1, he or she is eligible to receive benefits as of July 1.

■ MEDICARE ELIGIBILITY

Everyone eligible for SSDI also qualifies for Medicare. However, the beneficiary must wait 24 months from the date that benefits commence before coverage becomes effective.

During this qualifying period for Medicare, the recipient might be eligible for health insurance from a former employer or through a program offered by the state where the individual resides.

■ TRIAL WORK PERIOD

A person receiving SSDI benefits may be entitled to a trial work period, depending on his or her medical condition. The period used to determine the individual's ability to work is 9 months (to be performed during a 60-month consecutive period) while he or she is still drawing the full SSDI monthly benefit. After the 9 months of trial work, the beneficiary will lose the SSDI cash benefit if he or she earns more than $860 per month (as of 2006) from gainful employment.

Final note: The SSA is now in the process of reviewing the application process for SSDI and SSI. The goal is to bring clinical expertise into the process earlier and to limit the number of steps involved.

■ 5

SUPPLEMENTAL SECURITY INCOME

Supplemental Security Income (SSI) is a federal income support program administered by the Social Security Administration (SSA). It is a government benefit that provides a basic monthly income to individuals who are blind, disabled, or 65 years of age or older and who meet certain financial thresholds. Unlike Social Security Disability Insurance (SSDI), SSI is financed through general tax revenues, not taxes on the earnings of the applicant. Individuals can receive SSI even if they have never worked or would not otherwise qualify for Social Security. Its purpose is to provide cash to meet basic needs of food, clothing, and shelter.

Both disability and financial criteria need to be met for one to be eligible for SSI benefits. The disability must be a medically determinable mental or physical condition that is expected to have a duration of one year or longer or to result in death. Financial criteria include earned income (wages) and resource assets (bank accounts and other fluid assets).

To be eligible for SSI based on a medical condition, an applicant must have little or no income or resources. He or she must be a U.S. citizen, or meet the requirements for non-citizens, and must be a resident of one of the 50 states, the District of Columbia, or the Northern Mariana Islands. An applicant must be considered medically disabled and cannot be working, or working only in a job that is not considered substantial gainful activity.

■ FINANCIAL ELIGIBILITY

An individual applying to receive SSI cannot have assets that exceed $2,000. For a couple, the assets cannot have a value in excess of $3,000, even if only one individual is eligible for such benefits. In addition, an applicant's earned income may not be over $860 per month.

Certain assets are not included in determining SSI eligibility:

▪ The family home
▪ One automobile
▪ Burial plots for an individual applicant and his or her immediate family
▪ Burial funds up to $1,500
▪ Life insurance with a face value of $1,500 or less

Under SSI, income may be derived from cash or checks (their inclusion being dependent on the source of payment), as well as an array of assets (some of which may not even be reported on federal, state, or local income tax returns). Examples include

▪ Wages from work, whether in cash or in another form
▪ Net earnings from a business, if the applicant is self-employed
▪ The value of food, clothing, or shelter that someone gives the applicant or the amount of money given to that individual to help pay for such items
▪ Department of Veterans Affairs (VA) benefits
▪ Social Security benefits
▪ Annuities, pensions, workers' compensation, and unemployment insurance benefits
▪ Proceeds from life insurance policies
▪ Gifts and contributions
▪ Child support and alimony
▪ Inheritance in cash or property.

The following items are not considered income:

▪ Medical care and services
▪ Social services
▪ Receipts from the sale, exchange, or replacement of assets owned by the applicant
▪ Income tax refunds
▪ Earned income tax credit payments and proceeds of a loan
▪ Bills paid by someone else for items other than food, clothing, or shelter
▪ Replacement of lost or stolen income
▪ Home energy assistance

■ The first $20 of most income received in a month

■ The first $65 earned by the applicant above the $20 disregard and half of the amount earned over $65

■ Food stamps.

■ APPLICATION

Applicants can receive extensive information on SSI from the Social Security website: www.socialsecurity.gov. The website gives an overview of the application process and all of the steps involved. It also provides the opportunity for an online application, if preferred, as well as an estimate of an eligible individual's benefit amount.

One can also telephone SSA and arrange for an appointment to initiate the application process. The toll-free number is 1-800-772-1213. Representatives are available from 7:00 am to 7:00 pm each business day.

Application requires a number of documents. The more documentation the applicant has in advance, the more efficient the application process will be. Some of the items most likely to be requested include

■ Social Security card

■ Proof of age, documented by either the original or certified copy of the applicant's birth certificate

■ Proof of resources: bank accounts, life insurance, and cash

■ Proof of income: paycheck stubs or copies of payment received

■ Proof of living arrangements: rent or mortgage payments

■ Names, addresses, and telephone numbers of doctors, hospitals, and clinics

■ Documentation from employers, preferably by means of notarized statements, detailing work limitations due to the disability

Applications may also be submitted by an authorized representative but must also be signed by the applicant unless that individual is under the age of 18, is not physically able to sign, or lacks the mental competence to do so. In these cases, a court-appointed representative or other responsible person may sign on the applicant's behalf.

■ DISABILITY DETERMINATION

Federal statute provides that the same standard applies in determining disability for SSI and SSDI. Social Security uses a multi-step process in reaching this determination.

The process is primarily focused on diagnosis and on whether a person meets the criteria of listed impairments established by the SSA for that diagnosis. If disability cannot be determined on that basis, determination is based on "Residual Functional Capacity," what the individual can and cannot do in the workplace.

The applicant must be unable to engage in any substantial activity by reason of a medically determinable physical or mental impairment that is expected to last for a continuous period of not less than 12 months or result in death.

Questions that need to be answered regarding functioning include the following:

■ Does the applicant have a severe impairment?

■ Is the applicant not working or expected not to work?

■ Is the applicant engaged in any substantial gainful activity?

■ Is the applicant capable of performing relevant work?

The paperwork is the same as that required for someone establishing a disability when applying for SSDI benefits. The doctor's report, based on a recent examination, should include

1. Establishing a diagnosis of the illness or injury causing severe impairment of the work activity

2. Explaining how the individual meets the impairment criteria established by SSA for that diagnosis

3. Explaining the restriction of work capacity resulting from the diagnosed medical condition

4. Explaining whether the impairment will either result in death or be expected to last at least 12 months

■ APPEAL

If the SSA denies the initial application for SSI, the applicant has the right to appeal the denial of the claim. Although some changes in the appeal process are planned by the SSA in the future, the four steps of appeal currently include the following:

■ Reconsideration

■ Administrative law judge (ALJ) hearing

■ Appeals Council review

■ Federal court appeal

The claimant has 60 days from the time he or she receives a denial of the application to appeal the decision. Failure to file a timely appeal may result in a waiver of his or her rights for SSI benefits. An attorney may be retained at any level of the decision-making process.

It is not unusual for an initial application to be rejected. About 60 percent of original applications are denied. Many of these denials are overturned when appealed. Reconsideration is the first level of appeal, and about 20 percent of individuals win at this stage. The reversal rate can be over 50 percent when denials are appealed to the next level, which is before an ALJ. It is essential for anyone applying for SSI (or SSDI) to know these statistics, because the process is lengthy and rejection notices can be disheartening when issued without what appears to be a thorough consideration of the facts supporting the disability.

If the application is approved, the amount of the monthly SSI benefit is dependent on the recipient's income and living arrangements. As of 2006, the federal payment standard was $603 per month for an individual and $904 per month for a couple. In addition, 43 states provide supplemental payments to beneficiaries In most cases, SSI beneficiaries who work can deduct the costs of certain items they require for work (known as impairment-related work expenses), as well as transportation costs to and from the job, plus home and car modifications.

■ MEDICAID COVERAGE

Medicaid is a jointly funded federal-state health insurance program for low-income and needy people. It covers children, the aged, the blind, the disabled, and other people eligible to receive federally assisted income maintenance payments. The Center for Medicare & Medicaid Services oversees state administration of Medicaid. Title XIX of the Social Security Act authorizes Medicaid.

Thirty-two states and the District of Columbia authorize Medicaid eligibility to people eligible for SSI benefits. In these states, an SSI application also serves as a Medicaid application.

The following states use the same rules to decide eligibility for Medicaid as are used for SSI, but they require the claimant to file a separate application:

Alaska	Nebraska	Utah
Idaho	Nevada	Northern Mariana Islands
Kansas	Oregon	

The following states have their own eligibility criteria for Medicaid, which are different from the SSI rules. In these states, a claimant must also file a separate application for Medicaid:

Connecticut	Minnesota	Ohio
Hawaii	Missouri	Oklahoma
Illinois	New Hampshire	Virginia
Indiana	North Dakota	

Once an SSI or Medicaid application is approved, Medicaid coverage becomes effective immediately. There is no premium charged for coverage.

Should Counsel Be Retained During the Application Process?

As noted earlier for SSD benefits, no one likes to pay attorney fees. An individual might assume that the application will be swiftly approved after proof of diagnosis is submitted to the SSA. Unfortunately, however, it is not that simple. The SSA requires that an individual's condition has progressed to the point that he or she is functionally unable to engage in substantial gainful activity. Determination of benefits is based on meeting the criteria of impairment, not on diagnosis alone. In order to qualify for SSD benefits, the claimant must have a condition that is expected to last for a continuous period of not less than 12 months or to result in death. A person who wants to represent himself or herself must be confident that he or she has the skills to present the necessary proof to the SSA. Assuming that the applicant possesses the requisite expertise, will there be sufficient control of emotions if his or her integrity is questioned?

Another factor to consider is the slow pace set by the SSA in reaching a decision. For example, it generally takes three to five months for Social Security to gather all of the necessary evidence and to conduct a hearing before rendering a decision. A skillful attorney knows the roadblocks that are characteristic of the initial application process and how to avoid them.

It is fair to say that every case is different and that an attorney's role depends on the particular facts of the case. However, some of the things an attorney may do can be very time-consuming to the novice, including the following:

- Gather medical and other evidence.
- Analyze the case under the Social Security regulations.
- Refer the client to additional doctors whom the attorney has used previously and whose work he or she trusts.
- Send the client to a vocational expert for a report on his or her ability to work.
- Request subpoenas to ensure the presence of crucial witnesses or documents at the hearing.

In conclusion, an attorney is strongly recommended when an appeal is necessary. Whether one should be retained at the beginning of the application process depends on the ability and expertise of the applicant to negotiate this lengthy and cumbersome process. It is essential that, if an attorney is retained, he or she be knowledgeable of the SSI application process and preferably have experience representing individuals pursuing such claims. As with SSD benefits, the National Organization of Social Security Claimant Representatives (NOSSCR) is one resource for finding such an attorney.

■ ATTORNEY FEES

An attorney may charge and receive a fee for his or her services, but the SSA decides how much the fee will be. Generally, the maximum fee that will be authorized is 25 percent of the retroactive payment or $5,300, whichever is less. A representative cannot charge or receive more than the fee amount authorized. SSI differs from SSDI in that amounts cannot be withheld from an individual's SSI benefits to pay for attorney fees. SSI claimants are responsible for paying such fees directly to their attorneys.

6

SSDI AND SSI: THE APPLICATION PROCESS

Applicants can receive extensive information on the Social Security Disability Insurance (SSDI) and Social Security Income (SSI) programs from the Social Security website: www.socialsecurity.gov. The website gives an overview of the application process and all of the steps involved. It also provides the opportunity for an online application, if preferred. One can also telephone the Social Security Administration (SSA) and arrange for an appointment to initiate the application process. The toll-free number is 1-800-772-1213. Representatives are available from 7:00 am to 7:00 pm each business day.

Request the following items as you prepare to apply for benefits:

- The pamphlet titled "Disability Benefits"
- Social Security application
- Earnings and Benefits Estimate Statement

The person applying for SSDI or SSI needs to be aware that the procedure is not easy. The process can take six to eight months and requires the submission of a considerable amount of documentation to establish, among other things, proof of a disability and the applicant's work history.

Although there is no hard rule that the applicant must quit working before applying for benefits, any work is considered a factor by the SSA in establishing the presence of a disability. However, an application will be denied if the individual is earning more than $860 per month (as of 2006) in substantial gainful employment.

■ STEP 1: DESCRIPTION OF DISABILITY

This step can be initiated before the application is received. To prepare for completing the SSDI or SSI application, it is recommended that the applicant maintain, for at least one month, a log of daily activities that records the occurrence of symptoms such as the following:

- Visual difficulties
- Tremors
- Balance problems
- Memory loss
- Speech difficulties
- Weakness
- Bladder control
- Emotional distress
- Spasms
- Fatigue
- Sexual difficulties
- Numbness
- Short-term memory problems
- Concentration problems

It is also essential that the applicant keep track of his or her daily activities to help create a clear mental picture of the problems he or she faces, which in turn must be conveyed to the Social Security representative at the time of application. It is important to convey symptoms an individual has on his or her worst day, not the best day, and to be as comprehensive and descriptive as possible.

Following is a suggested self-survey containing the types of questions that need to be answered when one applies for SSDI or SSI.

Applicant Self-Survey to Prepare for SSDI or SSI Application

Name: _____

Date of Diagnosis: _____

I. GETTING OUT OF BED

1. How long does it take you to get up in the morning?
2. Do you require assistance to get up?

3. Once you are standing do you hold onto anything to steady yourself?

4. When walking to the bathroom, do you touch the walls? (This is called wall walking.) Why?

II. PERSONAL HYGIENE

1. If male, do you sit to urinate?

2. To shower, do you need assistance to get into the shower?

3. Do you sit or stand while showering?

4. If you stand while showering, do you lean against the shower wall?

5. Have you ever needed assistance in bathing?

6. Have you ever burned yourself because of the water temperature?

7. After you finish bathing, do you pause before you exit? How long?

8. Do you sit on the toilet seat to rest before you exit the bathroom?

9. To return to your room, do you use the walls for assistance?

III. DRESSING

1. Do you require assistance in selecting your clothes?

2. Do you dress in stages? For example, do you put on your shirt, and then pause before you select the next article of clothing?

3. Do you need assistance with buttons, snaps, or shoestrings?

4. Why do you need this assistance?

5. Do you need to rest after dressing? How long is this rest period?

6. How long does the entire dressing process take?

IV. MEAL PREPARATION

1. Has there been a change in the amount of food preparation that you can do independently?

2. What do you usually have for breakfast, lunch, and dinner?

3. Who prepares or assists you with meal preparation?

4. Why do you need assistance?

5. Have you ever fallen while preparing a meal?

6. Do dishes or pots and pans fall from your hands without warning?

7. Have you ever scalded yourself while making a meal?

8. Do you ever skip meals because you are too tired to prepare the food yourself?

9. Have you ever set off the smoke alarm because you forgot something on the stove?

10. Who does the shopping?

V. HOUSEHOLD DUTIES

1. Do you do your own personal shopping?

2. If not, who assists you?

3. Do you pay your own bills?

4. Do you take care of your banking needs?

5. Do you do your own laundry?

6. Do you drive?

7. Who assists you in your transportation needs?

8. Do you consider yourself a safe driver?

9. Who cleans your house?

VI. RECREATIONAL/SOCIAL

1. Before your symptoms began, what were your hobbies?

2. Have these hobbies changed?

3. What do you now do for entertainment?

4. How often do you visit your friends and family?

5. How often do friends and family come to visit you?

6. If you are a parent, how active are you with the children?

7. Has your interaction with the children changed?

You have explored your activities of daily living in great detail through this log. If there is any additional information you feel is important, that has not been addressed, please list it:

1._____

_____

_____

2._____

_____

_____

3._____

_____

■ STEP 2: WORK HISTORY

1. List the jobs held for the past 15 years:

Job title   Kind of business   Dates worked

_____   _____   _____

_____   _____   _____

_____   _____   _____

2. List basic duties of these jobs.
3. List any machines/tools or equipment you can use.
4. List any technical knowledge you may have.
5. Have you had supervisory responsibilities?

   Which do you do more of and how much of each in hours per day?
   Sitting _____
   Standing _____
   Walking _____
   (*Note:* The total of these three activities need to amount to eight hours.)

■ STEP 3: PHYSICIAN CONTACTS

Assemble the names and addresses, zip codes, and phone numbers of all the doctors and allied health professionals you have seen or who have treated you for your condition and/or its symptoms. Your list may include your:

- Neurologist or other medical specialist
- General practitioner
- Neuro-opthalmologist
- Urologist
- Physiatrist
- Psychiatric psychologist
- Occupational or physical therapist

■ STEP 4: FILING APPLICATION

1. Complete all forms as required.
2. Contact all doctors who have treated you to let them know that they will be requested to send your records to the Social Security Office. You may also want

to request a copy of these records for yourself. The submission of the doctor's report should be based on a recent examination and include:

– Establishing the diagnosis of the illness or injury that is causing severe impairment of the work activity;

– Explaining how you must meet the criteria of listed impairments as established by SSA for your diagnosis;

– Explaining the restriction on work capacity resulting from the diagnosed medical condition;

– Providing examples of what you can and cannot do; and

– Explaining if the impairment will either result in death or is expected to last at least 12 months.

▪ DETERMINATION

The SSA notifies claimants of their determination rating. This notification provides the date that the SSA determines as the onset of disability. There is a five-month waiting period from that date before payment of benefits begins.

7

EMPLOYEE RETIREMENT INCOME SECURITY ACT

In 1974 the federal government passed the Employee Retirement Income Security Act (ERISA) for the purpose of establishing uniform federal standards for pension and employee benefit plans, including health insurance plans. The primary purpose of adopting ERISA was to protect the solvency and security of employee pension plans. However, because the statute contained language preempting all state laws related to employee benefit plans, which could include health insurance plans, an unintended benefit was given to employers regarding health plans funded entirely by them (referred to as "self-funded plans").

In a self-funded plan, the employer, not an insurance company, collects all of the premiums and pays out all of the benefits. The employer is not purchasing a plan from an insurance company but is itself administering the plan. By doing so, the employer does not need to pay the administrative and overhead costs to the insurance company, and the self-funded plan is not regulated by state insurance regulations. On the other hand, the employer assumes all of the risks of the plan. It is estimated that over 60 percent of people who have health insurance provided by an employer or union are in self-funded plans. There is considerable variability in this figure among states.

Self-funded plans are established by employers or unions, but the actual administration or paperwork of the health plan may be processed by an outside entity, or "third party administrator" (TPA). Often the TPA of a self-funded plan is a well-known health insurer, such as Blue Cross/Blue Shield, which often leads covered individuals to believe they are insured by Blue Cross/Blue Shield when, in fact, they are insured by their employer's self-funded plan.

■ ERISA PREEMPTION

If an employer purchases a health insurance plan from a licensed insurance company, the insurer must comply with all applicable state insurance requirements. However, if the plan is funded entirely by the employer, ERISA preempts regulators from imposing such requirements on the employer. In other words, state legislatures and insurance regulators have the authority to impose requirements on insurers. ERISA preempts them from imposing health benefit plan requirements on employers.

The lack of state regulation limits the options available to those seeking accountability for medical decisions that result in harm—even if those decisions contradict the recommendation of the treating physician. Under ERISA, the family of a patient who is injured or dies as a result of a health plan decision must file an appeal in federal court and can recover only the cost of a denied benefit. ERISA prevents the family or patient from holding the plan accountable for the pain and suffering caused by the negligence. Therefore, if or when an individual chooses to file an appeal of a decision made by a health plan, it is very important to know whether the plan was self-funded. Although ERISA does not eliminate one's right to appeal an adverse decision, it does limit the scope of appeal rights.

ERISA plans are attractive to employers because they enable them to avoid most state regulations regarding insurance. State-mandated benefit laws have ballooned in recent years, from only 158 when ERISA was enacted to more than 1,000 today. These mandates often prescribe terms of group policies, including coverage requirements. ERISA plans avoid this regulation.

■ COURT DECISIONS

Since the mid-1990s, ERISA's preemption of state laws has weakened. Court decisions in 1995, 1997, and 1999 narrowed the scope of preemptions. In 1995, for example, in *New York State Conference of Blue Cross and Blue Shield v. Travelers Insurance Co.*, the Supreme Court held that New York could apply surcharges to the hospital bills of patients insured under self-funded plans. The decision represented the first major pullback by the Supreme Court from its long-standing reluctance to interpret the ERISA preemption standard expansively.

A more dramatic example of this turnaround was a federal district court decision of 1999. In this action, the insurer, an HMO, denied the plaintiff's teenage son psychiatric care, although he had tried to commit suicide on two occasions within a month. A week later, the boy committed suicide and the parents sued the HMO. Although the defendant raised ERISA as a defense, the court held that the claim fell outside the jurisdiction of ERISA because it involved medical negligence, not the improper denial of medical benefits. Earlier, this defense would have almost certainly been sufficient to dismiss the suit.

On June 12, 2000, the United States Supreme Court issued one of its most important decisions regarding ERISA protections and exemptions. In the case of *Pegram v. Herdrich*, Mrs. Herdrich claimed that the decision by her HMO physician, Dr. Pegram, to delay her medical treatment, which resulted in a burst appendix, was driven by the self-interest of the physician to increase her HMO incentive bonuses, thus violating her fiduciary duty under ERISA. (ERISA defines a fiduciary as one who administers the plan and acts solely in the interest of the plan's participants and beneficiaries.) If the Court agreed that HMO decisions were "fiduciary acts," Dr. Pegram's failure to act, causing medical harm, could be viewed as a breach of fiduciary duty and would allow the plaintiff to seek monetary damages in federal court.

The Supreme Court held that decisions made by plan doctors are not fiduciary acts within the meaning of ERISA. ERISA focuses on eligibility and benefit coverage and is not intended to govern medical treatment issues. Therefore, "treatment" decisions made by doctors that lead to claims of medical negligence do not come under federal law. Instead, state law should provide the insured with the appropriate remedies to hold HMOs accountable.

The importance of this decision is that it upheld the view that HMOs must be held accountable for harm to patients. Although not an issue for federal court, referring to applicable state law opened the way for expanded state legislation and regulation of ERISA plans.

Finally, on June 20, 2002, a divided (5 to 4) United States Supreme Court ruled, in the case of *Rush Prudential HMO, Inc. v. Moran*, that the Illinois Health Maintenance Organization Act is not preempted by ERISA. In this case, Moran had sought independent treatment review after her HMO denied coverage for surgery. The HMO was a self-funded plan regulated by ERISA, which does not require independent treatment review. The Illinois Act provides for independent medical review of certain denials for service, including disputes between the primary physician and the HMO regarding medical necessity. In deciding this case, the Court did not find any congressional intent for ERISA to preclude the Illinois statute and its application to the HMO.

■ LEGISLATIVE ACTIVITY

On the federal legislative level, there was an attempt to eliminate the ERISA preemption in 1999. The United States House of Representatives approved the Norwood-Dingle Bill, which would have permitted patients to hold managed care insurers legally accountable for a delay or denial of care that resulted in injury or death. Although the Senate chose to adopt a much weaker bill and the two houses were never able to reach a compromise on the legislation, it certainly brought attention to the desire of some legislators to weaken, if not eliminate, the preemption defense.

State legislative attempts to eliminate ERISA preemption, although not always successful, have focused on the following:

- The right to sue for medical malpractice
- The right to sue for violation of state patient protections
- Strengthening the internal appeals process
- Providing for independent medical review of certain denials of service, commonly referred to as "external review"

■ REGULATORY ACTIVITY

In November 2000 the Department of Labor issued regulations regarding ERISA plans and deadlines for notifying patients about coverage. These new regulations also required

- More time for the insured to appeal denial of health claims
- More information about the reasons for denial of the claim, and the criteria and rules applied by the plan
- The use of different decision makers to handle the initial determination and review of the decision
- Timely action for claimants receiving a course of treatment who face an early termination of benefits or have a need to extend treatment

ERISA continues to protect employers from having to comply with most state regulation and legislation regarding insurance. It enables multi-state companies to avoid state-based regulatory activity, and state departments of insurance have no jurisdiction over self-funded plans. Since the type of plan an employer offers determines appeal rights and protections available to the employee, it is important for everyone to determine whether his or her employer coverage is self-funded.

◼ 8

GRIEVANCES AND APPEALS

Every health plan must provide a procedure for the insured to challenge decisions of the insurer that are not in the insured person's favor. Such "adverse decisions" often involve denial of coverage for services that the insured and his or her doctor believe are medically necessary. The procedure to challenge decisions depends on whether the plan is a self-funded employer plan or one purchased from an insurance provider. States regulate the business of insurance, which includes health maintenance organizations (HMOs), preferred provider organizations (PPOs), or other types of managed care organizations (MCOs) that sell a health insurance policy to an individual, employer, or other purchaser. The federal government, pursuant to the federal statute ERISA (Employee Retirement Income Security Act; see Chapter 7), regulates private-sector employer health plans, including managed care plans that are administered by a private employer.

◼ ERISA PLANS

In a self-funded, or self-insured, group health plan, employers set aside funds to pay the health claims of their employees. By collecting the premiums, determining the benefits, and paying the claims, the employer assumes the total risk and financial responsibility of the employees' health insurance coverage. No insurance company is involved unless it is contracted to administer the paperwork. Approximately 65 percent of private-sector health plans are self-funded.

Self-funded plans evolved following passage in 1974 of the Employee Retirement Income Security Act (ERISA). Although this federal legislation focused on protecting the solvency and security of employee pension plans, an unintended benefit was the preemption of self-funded employer plans from state regulation and legislation.

Under ERISA, a self-funded employer plan must provide adequate notice in writing to any participant or beneficiary whose claim for benefits under the plan has been denied. The notice must explain the reasons for the denial and provide a reasonable opportunity for a full and fair review of the decision by the party that denied the claim.

Under ERISA, beneficiaries whose benefits have been wrongfully withheld are entitled only to equitable relief and monetary damages. In practical terms, the claimant's recovery is limited to the value of the denied service or the service itself. In other words, punitive damages may not be part of an award.

The federal regulations governing ERISA provide that plans subject to the statute allow 90 days from the date a claim is received for a response if the claim has been denied. The notice must explain the specific reasons for the denial and be written in a manner calculated to be understood by the claimant. A claimant is then allowed 60 days after receipt of the denial to request a review. A decision on the review must ordinarily be made within 60 days after the request for a review, unless special circumstances (such as the need to hold a hearing if the plan provides for one) require an extension of time.

ERISA exempts self-funded plans from state regulation. Although the states have been very innovative in using their regulatory authority to protect consumers during the grievance process, such reforms do not apply to the ERISA plans. For instance, current ERISA grievance and appeal rules do not distinguish between the types of claims for benefits under review (e.g., emergency vs. non-emergency services) or require external appeal procedures. ERISA requires only that plans provide a "meaningful" and "timely" procedure for hearing and resolving complaints. In other words, there is no federal standard that prescribes how complaint and appeal systems are to be structured and administered.

■ FULLY INSURED PLANS

Contrary to what the average consumer might consider to be fact, the states, rather than the federal government, have assumed the initiative of protecting patient rights in managed care. A state's commissioner of insurance is a source of specific information about patient protections in a state.

Some states have passed highly innovative laws to protect patient rights. For example, Maryland has enacted legislation that offers patients and health care providers state assistance in filing complaints with insurance companies. Other states are proposing laws on the types of grievance and appeals process that insurance companies must offer patients when benefits are denied.

The following examples describe typical state legislation impacting the grievance and appeal process:

▪ *Alaska.* Alaska adopted a patient's bill of rights that includes provision for a fair, prompt, and mutual dispute resolution process in the case of a dispute between a managed care company and the insured. This includes the availability of an external appeal process, the cost of which must be paid by the insurer.

▪ *California.* California amended its grievance procedure for denied claims to include the following provisions: The plan must specify the location(s) and telephone number(s) where grievances may be submitted. It must also furnish enrollees with written responses to grievances. If the grievance involves an adverse determination, the insurer's response must include all criteria and clinical reasons used in supporting the decision. The insurer must retain copies of all grievances and responses for at least five years. California also approved an external review procedure for experimental or investigational therapies pertaining to diseases that cause serious disability. The review must pertain to the denial of coverage of a specific drug, device, procedure, or other therapy that would have been covered except for the insurer's determination that the treatment is experimental or investigational.

▪ *Delaware.* Delaware enacted legislation providing, as a final step in the grievance process, a review of the denial by the State Independent Review Organization. The purpose of this agency is to review appealed issues of medical necessity, if requested by the insured or his or her representative, as an external process after all appeal alternatives have been exhausted.

▪ *Hawaii.* Hawaii's statute provides that, if the enrollee requests an expedited process and the circumstances meet the necessary standard, both internal and external appeals must be reviewed within 72 hours from the time they are submitted. Approval must be granted if the usual 45-day process would seriously jeopardize the "health, life, health status, or maximum function" of the insured.

The statute also mandates that a final internal determination will be subject to external review by a state panel, if requested by the enrollee. The review panel must consider the following factors in its deliberations:

— The terms of the managed care contract

— Whether the plan's medical director properly applied the medical necessity criteria

— All relevant medical records

— The clinical standards of the plan

— The information provided

— The attending physician's recommendation

— The generally accepted medical guidelines

▪ *Kentucky.* Kentucky's legislation provides that, in the event coverage is denied, in addition to stating the reason(s) for the decision, the plan must include instructions on how to file a request for review. In the case of a review, the only person who may conduct it and determine whether the initial finding should be affirmed or denied is a physician who did not participate in the initial review. The legislation also includes a procedure permitting the introduction of new clinical information that might be relevant in reversing the earlier denial if an external review is held.

■ *Maine*. State legislation established the right of enrollees to have their rejected claims assessed by an independent external review organization. Any decision rendered by this body is binding on the carrier. The carrier must also pay the expenses of the review.

■ *Maryland*. Maryland enacted legislation requiring that only physicians or a panel of medical experts may make grievance determinations. A panel is defined as a group of medical personnel, at least one of whom is a physician, who is either board certified or eligible in the same specialty as the service under review.

■ *Massachusetts*. Legislation was enacted requiring the insurer, when a grievance is filed, to maintain a formal internal process that provides for adequate consideration and timely resolution of proceedings, including

— A system for maintaining records for each grievance filed by an insured, and the responses of the insurer, for a period of seven years

— The inclusion in the determination notice of a statement describing the insurer's formal grievance process and the procedure to be followed in obtaining external review

— The insurer's toll-free number for assisting clients in resolving their grievances

— A written acknowledgment of receipt of the grievance within 15 days and a written resolution of each grievance within 30 days of receipt

— A procedure to accept grievances by telephone, in person, by mail, or by electronic means

A grievance not properly acted on by the insurer within the above time periods will be considered decided in favor of the insured.

■ *Michigan*. Michigan enacted legislation affecting the internal review process. In part, the statute provides the following:

— No request for external appeal may be made until the parties have exhausted the internal grievance process. However, if the medical condition of the insured is such that a delay in time would jeopardize the life or health of the individual, the external review may begin concurrently with the internal review process.

— The insured may begin the external review if the insurer has not been timely in issuing its determination.

— A description of both the standard and external appeals processes must be included in the notice of adverse determination. This description needs to state that the insured (or representative) has the right to furnish additional information for the organization's consideration.

■ *South Dakota.* South Dakota enacted legislation providing that resolution of grievances may involve the use of a mediation service.

■ *Virginia.* The state approved the following measures amending the independent review procedure used to consider claim denials:

— The legislation extended the number of working days in which the Bureau of Insurance must notify the claimant that his or her request for appeal is approved from 3 to 5 days.

— It extended the time frame in which the original review must be conducted from 5 to 10 working days.

— It extended the number of days in which medical records may be provided to the Bureau of Insurance from 10 to 20 days.

— It lowered the threshold for which a claimant can appeal a final adverse decision from $500 to $300.

■ CHALLENGING AN ADVERSE DECISION

If an adverse determination is made on a claim, it is important to review the health insurance contract carefully and become a smart and savvy consumer. If the contract clearly states that a particular service is not covered, it is doubtful that any number of appeals will reverse that. However, if the language is vague, refers only to "medical necessity," or indicates that the service has coverage, claimants should follow every level of the appeals process and do so as quickly as possible. The following steps should be taken to help resolve the problem:

■ It is imperative to organize an argument demonstrating the reasons why the denial letter was in error.

■ Assistance should be obtained from people who know how to structure a medical care appeal and who are on the insured's side. These include the employee's benefits manager, the claimant's physician, or personnel on the hospital staff. They can frequently help get the claims paid.

■ Claimants need to get the doctor on their side. This includes having the doctor write the insurer explaining the reasons why the claim should be approved. This letter should be included with the insured's letter of appeal.

■ It should be determined if the state has an ombudsman to assist in the negotiating process.

- The claimant should know (a) the medical reasons why the claim was denied; (b) the names of those involved in the decision denying the claim; and (c) whether these individuals have clinical expertise in the areas of medicine relevant to the medical problem.

- The claimant must find out how the plan's appeal process works. This means reading the plan contract carefully and reviewing the appeal process with the plan administrator, if necessary. For many complaints, the customer service representative may be able to resolve the problem over the phone.

- A second opinion should be secured or the claimant should obtain the names of other doctors recommending the type of treatment being requested.

- If the claimant is not satisfied with the representative's response, a supervisor should be requested immediately.

- If the case is not an emergency, the plan's administrative review board should reevaluate its initial determination. A letter of confirmation should be written, documenting which insurance representative agreed to send the matter to review, enclosing any other relevant material, and restating the action anticipated and the expectation that the review process will proceed expeditiously.

■ SAMPLE CLAIM/APPEAL LETTER

Date

Claim representative's name	Claimant's name
Representative's address	Claimant's address
City State ZIP	City State ZIP

Dear Claim Representative:

This letter serves as a request for reconsideration of payment of a denied claim related to the treatment of my medical condition.

As your records will show, I was diagnosed with _____ in (month and year). [Insert information regarding medical history, including previously attempted treatments and results.]

My neurologist (or physician), (name of doctor), wants me (to begin using the medication _____,) (to begin a regimen of physical therapy) (to undergo a [name of procedure]), which he or she believes is necessary in the proper treatment of (name of condition). He or she has prepared a letter explaining the medical necessity of the (drug) (physical therapy) (procedure) in the proper treatment of the illness, and that letter is enclosed with this reconsideration request.

Based on the above information, I would appreciate your reconsideration of coverage for these submitted charges.

Sincerely,

If reconsideration is denied, a follow-up letter should be sent requesting the following information:

- The medical reasons why the claim was denied
- The names and medical backgrounds of those individuals denying the claim
- Whether these individuals have clinical expertise in the particular chronic condition or disability and the extent of their experience
- Further steps of appeal available

■ STATE EXTERNAL REVIEW

As of 2004, 43 states and the District of Columbia had enacted legislation creating external review as a means of resolving disputes between health plans and consumers. Almost all of these states require that the claimant exhaust all of the health plan's internal grievance procedures before engaging in this external review process. However, once the internal review is completed, members have an option of having an independent review of their health plan's denial of coverage.

Although this means a long process, and often a cumbersome one, almost half of all denials are overturned when plan members do pursue this course of action. The rate of overturn varies by state. Currently, state external reviews apply only to members of insurance plans regulated by the state's Department of Insurance. Consumers covered by self-funded ERISA plans are not covered by state regulation and therefore need federal legislation for this option to be available to them.

9

HEALTH INSURANCE PORTABILITY AND ACCOUNTABILITY ACT

The Health Insurance Portability and Accountability Act (HIPAA) of 1996 is a federal law that provides health care consumers with basic rights designed to help them maintain their eligibility for group health benefits and protect their medical privacy. It is particularly helpful for people who have chronic illnesses, disability, or are otherwise considered "high risk." The law is intended to reduce barriers by guaranteeing that most workers, and their dependents, who change or lose their jobs will have continued access to health insurance coverage. It also fosters the development of state insurance programs for individuals ineligible for all other coverage due to their medical history.

HIPAA's protections apply to most health plans (whether insured or self-funded). However, the legislation does not apply to group health plans covering fewer than two participants, nor does it guarantee access to health insurance for anyone who is not currently covered by health insurance. HIPAA does not regulate premium rates.

◼ HIPAA'S ANTI-DISCRIMINATION PROTECTIONS

HIPAA guarantees that an individual cannot be denied enrollment in a group health plan on the basis of his or her health status, nor can he or she be charged a higher premium due to poor health. In other words, no one can be singled out and charged more or excluded from participating in an employer's group health plan, regardless of what health condition that individual may have. This goes a long way toward preserving fairness in the system.

■ PREEXISTING CONDITIONS

To understand the protections of HIPAA, one needs to understand three important concepts: "preexisting condition," "exclusion period," and "creditable coverage." By carefully defining these terms, HIPAA dramatically improves options for workers previously locked into a job for fear of losing their health insurance.

HIPAA defines a preexisting condition as "a condition (whether physical or mental) for which medical advice, diagnosis, care, or treatment was recommended or received within the six-month period ending on the enrollment date." Simply stated, it is any health condition for which one consulted a health care professional or received treatment (including prescribed medication) within the six-month period prior to enrollment in a new plan.

A preexisting condition exclusion is the period of time during which a health plan is not responsible for covering the costs of a preexisting condition. Very significantly, HIPAA does not ban exclusion periods. However, it limits them to 12 months for first-time enrollment in a health plan and 18 months for late enrollment (enrollment after or between open enrollment periods).

■ CREDITABLE COVERAGE

Creditable coverage gives an individual (or dependent) credit for the amount of time he or she is insured in one group health plan (called prior coverage) and applies it to the preexisting condition exclusion period of a new plan. This means that someone can join a new group plan without a waiting period for coverage of a preexisting condition and with no exclusion for costs associated with care for that preexisting condition, as long as he or she has had 12 months of creditable coverage. This is what is meant by "portability" of coverage.

Creditable coverage includes prior coverage from group health plans, individual policies, union and association plans, state high-risk pools, Medicare, Medicaid, military health plans, the Indian Health Service, health plans of the Peace Corps, public health plans of foreign nations, and federal employee health plans. However, many student plans, catastrophic or disease-specific policies, private disability policies, "temporary" health policies, and dental or vision policies are not considered creditable coverage under HIPAA.

There is one other special requirement that must be met when it comes to the portability of creditable coverage. Prior coverage is not considered creditable if there is a gap of 63 or more consecutive days without coverage.

Here are three scenarios to illustrate how HIPAA protections work.

Marian was diagnosed with MS while she was working for ABC Corporation and was insured by ABC's group health plan. After three years with ABC, she took a job with DEF International and enrolled in its group health plan. Marian had a gap of just nine days between her ABC coverage and the start date of DEF's group plan. DEF's plan had a policy of excluding preexisting conditions for the first 12 months, but HIPPA allowed her to apply her prior coverage from ABC to DEF's preexisting condition exclusion period. Her MS expenses were covered right away.

Annette, who has Parkinson's disease, was covered by husband Greg's group health plan for the 10 months he worked for ABC. Then he was laid off. They did not elect COBRA because they could not afford the premiums. Greg got a new job with XYZ that offered health benefits to its workers and dependents. He enrolled in the XYZ plan and had only a 24-day gap in coverage. The new plan had a 12-month preexisting condition exclusion. However, HIPAA enabled Greg to deduct the 10 months of Annette's prior coverage from the 12-month exclusion period. They had to absorb uncovered costs related to her Parkinson's (the "preexisting condition") for only 2 months until the exclusion period was finished.

Janet has lupus and lost her job and health benefits when her employer downsized. She did not elect COBRA because of the expense. Janet found another job, three months later, that had a group health plan, and she enrolled in the plan right away. However, because more than 63 days had elapsed between the two plans, Janet did not get any credit for her prior coverage. She had no insurance for lupus-related health care expenses for a full year. However, other medical costs that Janet incurred during that period, which were unrelated to lupus, were covered by her new plan.

If Janet had elected COBRA, she would have remained covered until her new group coverage took over. Therefore, since COBRA is creditable coverage, it is important for people with expensive health conditions to elect their COBRA benefits so that they will not be without coverage for 63 days or more and be ineligible for HIPAA protections.

Demonstrating Prior Coverage

When a covered employee, spouse, or covered dependent leaves a plan, he or she must be given a Certificate of Coverage indicating the amount of time each individual had coverage. If one has a preexisting condition, this certificate is the proof of prior coverage that can be applied toward a preexisting condition exclusion period. The law requires all health plans to provide these certificates within a "reasonable" time. One should expect it shortly after leaving the job or at the end of the COBRA period (if elected).

Guaranteeing HIPAA Coverage

When considering the purchase of any health insurance policy, ask if it would be considered "creditable coverage" under HIPAA. Consult your employer, health plan administrator, or state department of health for more details about HIPAA protections.

■ HIPAA PROVISIONS FOR INDIVIDUAL INSURANCE

Most of the portability provisions in HIPAA provide assistance for people transitioning from one group health plan to another ("group to group"). Less attention was given to the "individual insurance market," whose regulation had traditionally been left to state lawmakers.

However, HIPAA does include incentives for states to reduce the barriers to coverage for the self-employed and others not eligible for group coverage. A number of approaches are currently in place, including high-risk pools (see Chapter 13), "guarantee issue" rules for individual insurance plans statewide, and "conversion policies" that enable former group members to convert their former coverage into an individual plan.

HIPAA also establishes a federal "fallback" for individuals living in states without a viable mechanism for individual coverage .It requires individual health plans to accept consumers on a guarantee issue basis if they lose group coverage and meet the following criteria:

1. Have had prior medical coverage for 18 consecutive months, with the most recent coverage being a group plan
2. Have no other coverage
3. Have not lost prior coverage as a result of fraud or nonpayment of premium
4. Have applied no later than 62 days after loss of the last coverage
5. Are ineligible for, or have exhausted, other coverage options, such as COBRA, state continuation requirements ("mini-COBRA"), Medicare, Medicaid, or other group coverage

■ LONG-TERM CARE INSURANCE

The tax consequences of long-term care insurance have also been modified under HIPAA. The new provision ensures that the tax treatment for private long-term care insurance is the same as for major medical coverage.

Once a plan becomes tax qualified, the taxpayer may claim "qualified long-term care insurance premiums" and unreimbursed long-term care medical expenses as itemized medical deductions on Schedule A, Form 1040 if this figure, along with other deductible medical expenses, exceeds 7.5 percent of adjusted gross income.

To benefit under the policy, the individual claiming these long-term expenses must be chronically ill, which is defined as being (1) unable to perform at least two activities of daily living (e.g., eating, toileting, continence) without special assistance from another person for a period of at least 90 days, or (2) requiring substantial supervision to protect that individual from threats to health and safety due to severe cognitive impairment. A health care practitioner is the one called upon to make this determination.

The expenses that qualify for tax deductions include monies expended on necessary diagnostic, preventive, therapeutic, curing, and rehabilitative services.

▪ HEALTH CARE FRAUD

A major issue addressed by HIPAA was the adoption of measures designed to fight health care fraud. Demonstrating its commitment, Congress appropriated millions of dollars to carry out its agenda and established annual increases in the appropriation. Major features of the health care fraud section of HIPAA include the following:

▪ The strengthening of the mandate given to the Office of Inspector General (OIG), the FBI, and the Department of Justice to enable those agencies to investigate all health care fraud, regardless of the source of payment. In addition, the Department of Justice is given the authority to subpoena records relating to health care fraud, regardless of the payer source.

▪ The enactment of the crime of "health care fraud," making it illegal for anyone to "knowingly and willfully execute a scheme to defraud any health care benefit program, in connection with the delivery of or payment for health care benefits, or to obtain, by means of false representations, any of the property of a health care benefit program." The crime is premised on the existing statutory provisions of mail and wire fraud, although the penalties under the health care fraud section are more extensive and the crime is targeted to the health care business. The crime does not require use of the United States mail or interstate wire system, but instead involves any efforts to defraud health care payers, no matter how the fraud is conducted.

▪ The creation of the Medicare Integrity Program, through which the Secretary of Health and Human Services enters into contracts with private-sector concerns to carry out Medicare investigative activities.

■ The establishment of a program designed to encourage Medicare beneficiaries to report fraud and authorizing the payment of rewards for furnishing information.

■ The creation of a department in the OIG with the authority to issue advisory opinions on the permissibility of certain business plans.

■ The enactment of a new civil money penalty that imposes fines against physicians who falsely certify home health care for individuals not requiring this care.

■ The creation of a database to maintain information on providers that have been sanctioned for health care fraud and abuse. The database is limited to "final adverse actions," a phrase that specifically excludes "settlements in which no findings of liability have been made."

■ The establishment of a new crime for the obstruction of investigations involving federal health care offenses. It applies to any health care investigation and process by a criminal investigator, which means any health care fraud investigator for a prosecutorial agency.

■ PRIVACY

HIPAA legislation also establishes privacy rules to give individuals more control over their health information. It requires health plans and providers to have written privacy procedures, to train employees involved in handling protected information, and to establish a grievance procedure. Providers with direct treatment relationships are required to make a good-faith effort to obtain an individual's written acknowledgment that he or she is aware of the provider's privacy practices.

■ SUMMARY

As should be readily apparent, HIPAA has changed the face of health insurance for individuals with preexisting conditions. Although portability does not mean that people will carry the same health insurance plan from job to job, it does mean that individuals with preexisting conditions will not lose coverage because of a change in jobs (assuming that the new employer provides coverage) or health plans. It also addresses an issue requiring the nation's immediate attention, namely, health care fraud.

The practical impact is that no enrollment may be delayed or otherwise conditioned on a health-related factor. This would prohibit the prior practice of requiring a new employee to furnish satisfactory evidence of good health as a condition for enrollment in the employer's plan. Health-related factors included medical condition, claims experience, receipt of medical care, medical history, genetic information, and evidence of insurability.

10

CONSOLIDATED OMNIBUS BUDGET RECONCILIATION ACT OF 1985

In 1985 the United States Congress enacted legislation, commonly referred to as COBRA (the Consolidated Omnibus Budget Reconciliation Act), to provide a vital health plan bridge for qualified workers and their spouses and dependent children who might otherwise lose their health insurance coverage. Its security and breadth is seen as a much needed safety net for families in the midst of crises such as unemployment, divorce, or death. These crises are referred to as "qualifying events."

COBRA requires employers that provide group health coverage to offer employees the opportunity to purchase continuation of that group coverage at the group plan rate if their employment is being terminated or under other special circumstances. Premiums must be paid fully by the former employee, as the employer would no longer contribute, but the rate for coverage would almost certainly be less costly than the purchase of an individual policy.

COBRA generally covers health plans of employers with 20 or more employees who worked at least 50 percent of the days in the previous calendar year. When used in this context, the term "employee" includes individuals working full-time and part-time, as well as those who are self-employed, provided they are eligible to participate in the employer health plan on the day before a qualifying event.

The coverage is broad, applying to plans in both the private sector and those established for individuals employed by state or local government. The federal government and certain church-related organizations are not subject to COBRA. As for those employers subject to the statute, COBRA benefits must be offered to employees benefiting from coverage, as well as to spouses and dependents covered under the plan.

However, the law stipulates that COBRA does not extend to the following individuals:

- An employee who is not yet eligible for the employer's group health plan (e.g., a new or part-time employee)
- An employee whose employment was terminated due to gross misconduct
- An eligible employee who declined coverage
- An individual who is enrolled for benefits under Medicare

■ QUALIFYING EVENTS

The continuation of insurance coverage, which is at the heart of COBRA, is determined by what is called a "qualifying event": an occurrence that triggers the insured's protection under COBRA. Whether a circumstance is defined as a qualifying event is contingent on the status of the insured. The rules are also dependent on whether the insured is the employee, the spouse of the employee, or his or her dependent. The following are qualifying events for employees:

- Voluntary or involuntary termination of employment for reasons other than gross misconduct
- A reduction in the number of hours, thus changing the status of the insured to part-time, thereby eliminating his or her eligibility

The following are qualifying events for spouses:

- Voluntary or involuntary termination of the covered employee's employment for any reasons other than gross misconduct
- A reduction in the number of hours worked by the covered employee
- The covered employee becoming entitled to Medicare
- Divorce or legal separation of the covered employee
- Death of the covered employee

The qualifying events for dependent children are the same as for the spouse, with the following addition:

- Loss of dependent child status under the plan rules

Depending on the type of event and the beneficiary, coverage could continue for 18, 29, or 36 months after the date of the event of the coverage loss. The law provides as follows:

Qualifying Event	Coverage	Beneficiary
Termination Reduced hours	18 months[1]	Employee Spouse Dependent child
Employee enrolls in Medicare; or divorce, legal separation, or death of the covered employee	36 months	Spouse Dependent child
Loss of dependent child status	36 months	Dependent child

[1]If a qualified beneficiary is determined under Title II or XVI of the Social Security Act to have been disabled within the first 60 days of COBRA coverage, then the qualified beneficiary and all qualified beneficiaries in his or her family may be able to extend COBRA continuation coverage for an additional 11 months. Notice of the determination must be given to the plan administrator within 60 days of the date of determination and before the end of the 18-month COBRA continuation period.

Coverage begins on the date that coverage would otherwise have been lost by reason of a qualifying event and ends when the following occurs:

■ The last day of maximum coverage is reached.

■ Premiums are not paid on a timely basis.

■ The employer ceases to maintain a group health plan.

■ A beneficiary is entitled to Medicare benefits.

■ Coverage is obtained with another employer group health plan that does not contain any exclusion or limitation with respect to a preexisting condition.

Although COBRA specifies certain maximum periods of time that continued health coverage must be offered to qualified beneficiaries, it does not prohibit plans from offering continuation of health coverage that goes beyond the COBRA periods.

■ COVERED BENEFITS

Identical Coverage Benefit

Qualified beneficiaries (individuals receiving coverage based on COBRA) must be offered benefits identical to those the individual received immediately before qualifying for continuation coverage. The coverage continuation rules apply to any type of employer-provided group health plan, whether insured or self-insured, funded or self-funded. Health care for this purpose includes indemnity, health maintenance organization (HMO), and preferred provider organization (PPO) plans.

Under COBRA, a group health plan is ordinarily defined as a plan that provides medical benefits for the employer's own employees and their dependents through insurance or another mechanism such as a trust, HMO, self-funded pay-as-you-go program, reimbursement, or a combination of these. Medical benefits provided under the terms of the plan and available to COBRA beneficiaries may include the following:

- Inpatient and outpatient hospital care
- Physician care
- Surgery and other major medical benefits
- Prescription drugs
- Any other medical benefits, such as dental and vision care

Neither life nor disability insurance is covered under COBRA.

Deductibles and Co-Insurance

The COBRA statute also requires that deductibles and co-insurance amounts for qualified beneficiaries not be greater than those for active employees.

Plan Options

If the plan provides options to covered employees, those options must be made available to qualified beneficiaries. An example of an option is the right of the employee to convert his or her group coverage to individual health insurance without regard to preexisting conditions and without having to undergo a medical examination or otherwise demonstrate proof of insurability.

Plan Limitations

The coverage provided to qualified beneficiaries must have the same benefit limits and limits on out-of-pocket expenses that are made available to covered employees. Moreover, like deductibles, any amounts already credited to the limits prior to a qualifying event are carried forward into the continuation coverage period.

Core and Non-Core Benefits

A qualified beneficiary, during the period he or she was covered while employed, might have been insured under a policy providing both core and non-core benefits. Core coverage includes all of the health benefits available to the insured individual other than dental and vision benefits, which are the only types of coverage defined as non-core.

Under law, qualified beneficiaries may limit coverage to core benefits alone, even if they had both types of coverage while employed. In other words, the insurer or employer is prevented from forcing unwanted coverage and a higher premium on the COBRA-qualified beneficiary.

■ NOTICE AND ELECTION PROCEDURES

Notice by the Employer

An initial notice describing COBRA rights must be furnished to qualified beneficiaries (insured employees and their covered spouses and dependents) when the plan becomes subject to the provisions of COBRA, or to new employees and their covered spouses and dependents ,when they join the plan.

If the health plan is self-insured, and the employer is not the plan administrator, the employer must provide notice to the outside administrator within 30 days from the date coverage ceases or the date of the following qualifying event:

■ Death of the covered employee

■ Termination of the covered employee for reasons other than gross misconduct

■ The covered employee becoming entitled to Medicare

■ The employer's bankruptcy

The administrator, in turn, has 14 days to notify qualified beneficiaries of their COBRA rights due to the occurrence of a qualifying event.

Notice by the Employee

An employee or spouse must notify the plan administrator (or employer, if there is no administrator) of the occurrence of any of the following:

■ Divorce

■ Legal separation

▪ Cessation of dependent's eligibility (i.e., loss of dependency status)

▪ Death of the employee

Notice must be given within 60 days of the qualifying event, or the date the qualified beneficiary would lose coverage as a result of the event, whichever is later. The group plan is not obligated to offer the qualified beneficiary the opportunity to elect COBRA coverage if the covered employee or qualified beneficiary fails to make the required notification.

Notice by Disabled Beneficiaries

A disabled beneficiary is entitled to an extra 11 months of continuation coverage in addition to the 18 months provided by law, if the Social Security Administration (SSA) determines that there was disability within the first 60 days of COBRA coverage. To qualify, disabled beneficiaries must notify the plan administrator of their disability within 60 days of their disability determination and before the end of the 18-month COBRA continuation period.

Election

Qualified beneficiaries are given a 60-day period to elect or reject coverage. This period is measured from the coverage loss date or the date the COBRA election notice is provided, whichever is later.

Although each qualified beneficiary may independently elect coverage, a covered employee or the employee's spouse may elect coverage for all of the other qualified beneficiaries. A parent or legal guardian may also elect on behalf of a minor child. The law further allows a qualified beneficiary to elect coverage after waiving it if the election is made within the 60-day period.

▪ COST OF COVERAGE

Beneficiaries are required to pay the entire premium for coverage. The premium cannot exceed 102 percent of the cost of the plan to similarly situated individuals who have not incurred a qualifying event. This includes both the portion paid by employees and any portion paid by the employer before the qualifying event, plus 2 percent for administrative costs. When an employee gets extended coverage due to a disability, the premium charged for months 18 through 29 may be increased to 150 percent of the cost of the plan.

Except for the initial payment, federal law states that payment of a premium is considered timely if made within 30 days after the due date, unless a longer due date is permitted in the plan. Some COBRA plan administrators send payment notices, or invoices, to qualified beneficiaries, although a beneficiary is responsible for timely payment with or without an invoice.

Some plans require monthly payments, and others allow for payment on a quarterly basis. Federal law provides that COBRA coverage can be canceled if premium payments are not made within the 30-day cycle. As for the first payment, a qualified beneficiary has 45 days, measured from the date of the COBRA election, to pay the premium.

▪ CERTIFICATE OF COVERAGE

To ensure that a plan or insurer will recognize an individual's prior health coverage, HIPAA requires the issuance of a Certificate of Coverage. This certificate enables an individual to provide evidence of prior creditable coverage, in order to reduce or completely avoid any preexisting condition exclusion that would otherwise limit the coverage of a subsequent group or individual health plan. Because the certificate of coverage provides important protections, especially for those with preexisting conditions, it should be kept with other important insurance and legal documents.

Legislation requires that plans and issuers furnish certificates automatically to the following:

▪ An individual entitled to elect COBRA continuation coverage at a time no later than when a notice is required to be provided for a qualifying event under COBRA

▪ An individual who has elected COBRA continuation coverage, either within a reasonable time after a plan learns that COBRA continuation coverage ceased or, if applicable, within a reasonable time after the individual's grace period for the payment of COBRA premiums ends

A certificate must always be provided at the written request of the participant, the covered spouse, or any of the insured dependents, provided that this request is made within 24 months after the individual loses coverage under the plan. When a certificate is requested, it must disclose each period of continuous coverage.

If the insured has more than 18 months of uninterrupted coverage, the certificate may simply show 18 months of creditable coverage without mentioning dates. If coverage is less than 18 months, the certificate must disclose the dates that coverage commenced and ended. In any case, the certificate needs to disclose only the most recent period of continuous coverage without a 63-day break.

If a qualified beneficiary is determined under Title II or XVI of the Social Security Act to have been disabled within the first 60 days of COBRA coverage, the qualified beneficiary and all qualified beneficiaries in his or her family may be able to extend COBRA continuation coverage for an additional 11 months. Notice of the determination must be given to the plan administrator within 60 days of the date of determination and before the end of the 18-month COBRA continuation period.

11

STATE "MINI-COBRA" LAWS

The Consolidated Omnibus Budget Reconciliation Act of 1985 (COBRA) provides for an individual who is working, has group health insurance, and voluntarily resigns from a job or is terminated for any reason other than gross misconduct, to be given the right to continue the coverage for up to 18 months at his or her expense. This period of coverage is extended to 29 months if the insured is determined to have been disabled within 60 days of becoming eligible for COBRA, and to 36 months for the spouse and dependent children of a covered employee if the employee becomes eligible through the death or divorce of the employee or if the child loses his or her dependent status under the terms of the plan.

In general, three groups of people qualify for COBRA benefits: employees or former employees in private business, their spouses, and their dependent children. Eligibility also extends to workers in state and local government and to workers classified as independent contractors. However, the law exempts an employer with fewer than 20 employees, federal government employers, and certain church-related organizations.

Fortunately, a number of states have taken the initiative of adopting legislation, referred to as "mini-COBRA" laws, or "continuation of coverage" laws, that extends many of the benefits of COBRA to state residents who do not qualify under the federal law.

Notwithstanding state legislation, the question is still raised of whether a self-funded plan, not qualifying for COBRA and limited under the federal ERISA law, would be subject to a state's mini-COBRA statute. Some states adopt the view that a self-funded plan under ERISA preempts a mini-COBRA law. Other states take the opposite stand. Because of this conflict, it is suggested that clients participating in self-funded plans check with their state's insurance department to find out (a) if the state has a mini-COBRA statute and (b) if so, whether coverage could be continued, notwithstanding ERISA.

■ MINI-COBRA OR CONTINUATION OF COVERAGE LAWS CURRENTLY IN EFFECT IN 40 STATES

Arkansas: Under state law, continuation of an employee's group coverage includes the following features:

■ An individual insured through an employer-based group health plan has the right to continue his or her coverage for up to 120 days due to termination of employment.

■ Death, divorce, or legal separation of the employee also triggers up to 120 days of continued coverage for the covered spouse and dependent.

■ The employee must have been insured for a period of at least three months immediately prior to the event triggering the continuation.

California: California has a continuation policy providing limited benefits. The legislation includes the following benefits:

■ An insured in a group health plan has the right to continue his or her health coverage for up to 18 months, if eligible before 1/1/03, or up to 36 months, if eligible after 1/1/03.

■ Continuation of coverage is also extended to dependents who were insured under the previous policy.

■ Coverage ceases when the insured obtains other group insurance, even if the terms of the plan are less substantive.

Colorado: Colorado provides a program similar to COBRA for insured groups not subject to that federal law. Its features include the following:

■ Termination of employment of the insured or his or her death, divorce, or legal separation triggers up to 18 months of continued coverage.

■ The employee must be insured under the employer-based group policy for at least 6 months immediately prior to termination.

■ Continuation is not available to employees and dependents covered under Medicare or Medicaid.

Connecticut: Under state law, continuation of an employer's group health coverage includes the following benefits:

■ The employee, spouse, and dependents have the right to continue their coverage for a period of up to 18 months if the qualifying event is termination of employment.

■ Connecticut allows up to 156 weeks (three years) of continuation following the death, divorce, or legal separation of the covered employee.

■ State law requires the employer to send "Notices of Option" within 10 days (not 14 or 44 days, as permitted under COBRA) to continue the group policy to the covered employee, dependents, and qualified beneficiaries if the loss of coverage is from termination, death, or total disability.

■ State law may not be used if COBRA coverage is elected.

Florida: For insured groups not subject to COBRA, Florida has a continuation statute that parallels some of the provisions of the federal law. Features of this legislation include the following:

■ An individual insured through an employer-based group health plan has the right to continue his or her coverage for up to 18 months if employment is terminated or hours of work are reduced.

■ Termination may not be due to the gross misconduct of the employee.

■ Death, divorce, or legal separation of the employee also triggers up to 18 months of continued coverage for the insured spouse and dependents.

■ A qualified beneficiary (defined as the covered employee, spouse, or dependent child) is entitled to an additional 11 months of coverage if he or she becomes disabled, as determined by the SSA, and notification of same is provided to the employer within 60 days from the date of determination and prior to the end of the 18-month continuation period.

Georgia: Georgia has a continuation program that provides limited benefits. The legislation includes the following features:

■ An insured has the right to continue his or her health coverage for up to 90 days due to termination of employment.

■ The insured must be covered under the plan for a period of at least six months immediately preceding the termination.

■ Following the 90-day extension, the insured has the option to convert the policy to individual coverage.

Illinois: For insured groups not eligible for COBRA, Illinois has a continuation statute providing limited benefits. The legislation includes the following features:

■ A qualifying event includes the termination of the insured's employment (unless termination was due to theft or commission of a work-related felony) as well as divorce, death, legal separation, or annulment.

■ Continuation of insurance must be offered to employer groups of any size, provided that the insured was covered for three continuous months before a qualifying event.

■ Coverage during continuation must be the same as provided in the group plan, but it need not include extra benefits such as prescription drugs.

■ Coverage continues for a maximum of nine months, and premiums may not exceed the group rate.

Iowa: Iowa provides a program similar to COBRA for an individual insured in a group health plan by an employer with 2 to 19 employees. The legislation includes the following benefits:

■ The insured must be covered under the policy for a period of at least three months immediately preceding termination of employment.

■ Termination of employment or membership in the group policy triggers up to nine months of continuation coverage.

■ The insured's death, divorce, legal separation, or annulment also triggers nine months of continuation coverage for the covered spouse or legal dependent.

■ Coverage ceases if the insured becomes eligible for Medicare or another group plan.

Kansas: Under state law, individuals working in concerns with 2 to 19 employees are entitled to benefits similar to COBRA. The statute includes the following features:

■ An insured in a group has the right to continue his or her health coverage for up to six months following termination of employment.

■ The insured's death, divorce, legal separation, or annulment also triggers six months of continuation coverage for the covered spouse or legal dependent.

■ The insured must be covered under the group policy at least three months immediately preceding a qualifying event.

■ Continuation is not available to someone eligible for Medicare.

Kentucky: Under state law, individuals working in concerns with 2 to 19 employees are entitled to benefits similar to COBRA. The statute includes the following features:

■ The legislation applies to an individual who has been covered under the employer-based group policy for at least three months immediately preceding the event triggering the continuation.

■ Continuation of coverage is triggered by the termination of the individual's employment. Divorce, death, or legal separation of the employee also triggers continuation for the spouse and dependent.

■ The extension of insurance is for a period of 18 months.

■ Continuation is not available to an individual who is eligible for Medicare or could be covered under another group plan.

Louisiana: This state has enacted legislation with COBRA-like benefits to individuals working in concerns with 2 to 19 employees. The law includes the following features:

■ An individual who has been insured under a group health policy through his or her employer and has been continuously employed for at least three months prior to termination is entitled to up to 12 months of continued coverage.

■ The insured has 90 days (not just 60 days, as provided by COBRA) to exercise this option, and premiums may not exceed the amounts charged under the group plan.

Maine: Under state law, insured groups are entitled to limited benefits. The statute includes the following features:

■ Coverage continues for up to six months if termination is based on the insured's layoff or a work-related condition.

■ Continuation of coverage may be as long as 12 months if the employee is totally disabled at the time of election.

Maryland: The state has a statute that is similar to COBRA but not as broad. The legislation includes the following benefits:

■ The law provides continuation of coverage for involuntarily laid-off employees and their dependents.

■ Continued coverage will be for a term of up to 18 months if the insured was covered for at least 30 days before termination.

■ The insurer may charge a premium of up to 102 percent of the group rate.

Massachusetts: Under state law, individuals in insured employer group plans are entitled to continuation similar to COBRA. The legislation includes the following features:

■ Coverage can continue up to 36 months, depending on the qualifying event.

■ The premium on the continuation policy may not exceed the amount charged for the group coverage.

■ Coverage ceases when the insured becomes eligible for another group plan.

Minnesota: In Minnesota, the statute providing continuation of the employer-based group policy includes the following features:

■ Rules are similar to COBRA for small employers (2 to 19 employees) in that the employee has the right to continue health coverage for up to 18 months from the time employment ends.

■ The premium for the new policy may not exceed 102 percent of the group rate.

■ If an insured individual becomes totally disabled while employed, the employer may not terminate or suspend coverage on the grounds that the employee is no longer working. The employee's coverage cannot be terminated as long as the premium is paid, which may be as much as 102 percent of the amount charged for the group plan (the figure of 102 percent, common in many states but greater for some, allows for a 2 percent administration fee).

■ Coverage ceases when the insured becomes covered under another group policy.

Mississippi: State continuation policy is limited and includes the following features:

■ An insured in a group health plan has the right to continue his or her health coverage for up to 12 months after termination of employment.

■ The insured must have been covered under the group policy for at least three months immediately preceding the qualifying event.

■ Coverage under this provision does not extend to individuals entitled to another group plan, provided that plan does not contain a provision excluding coverage because of a preexisting condition.

Missouri: Under state law, continuation of an employee's group coverage includes the following features:

■ A person working for a concern that employs 2 to 19 individuals and is in a fully insured group health plan has the right to continue health coverage for nine months after his or her job ends.

■ The employee must have been insured for a period of at least three months immediately prior to the qualifying event (termination of employment, death, divorce, or legal separation).

■ Coverage continuation will be for a period of nine months.

Nebraska: Under state law, continuation of an employee's group coverage includes the following features:

■ If the employee is covered under a group health plan and terminated from employment, the insurance will continue for a period of six months on a monthly renewal basis.

■ For insured groups not subject to COBRA, death of the employee entitles dependents to up to one year of coverage.

■ If coverage is continued, the premium charged may not exceed 102 percent of the group rate.

Nevada: State law provides a program similar to COBRA for an individual insured in a group health plan by an employer with 2 to 19 employees. The legislation includes the following features:

■ If the employee is terminated for any reason other than gross misconduct, coverage will be extended for 18 months.

■ In the case of the termination (other than for gross misconduct), death, divorce, or legal separation of the employee, the extension for a covered spouse or dependent child will be 36 months.

■ These extensions do not apply to an individual who voluntarily resigns.

■ The employee, spouse, or dependent child must be insured for a period of at least 12 months immediately preceding the termination of coverage.

■ The amount charged for the continuation policy may not exceed 125 percent of the group rate.

New Hampshire: State law provides a program similar to COBRA. The legislation contains the following features:

■ The legislation applies to an individual who has been employed for at least six months. It also extends to the insured's spouse or dependent, if covered under the policy.

■ Continuation of coverage is triggered by the termination of the individual's employment. Divorce or legal separation also triggers continuation.

■ The extension of insurance will be for a period of 18 months, except when the employee becomes disabled at any time during the first 60 days of coverage under this statute. In such case, the term of coverage will be 29 months.

■ The premium may not exceed 102 percent of the amount charged for the group policy.

New Jersey: State law establishes a COBRA-like policy for individuals who had been covered under employer-based group health plans and are no longer working. The features of this legislation include the following:

▪ If an employee who has group coverage is terminated, is transferred to part-time status, or ends employment, he or she is given the option of continuing the insurance.

▪ The continued coverage will have a term of 18 months.

▪ The premium on the new coverage may not exceed 102 percent of the premium paid for covered persons who are similarly situated.

▪ Coverage under state continuation will cease if one of the following occurs:
  — The employer chooses not to provide health benefits to any employees.
  — The employee fails to make payment of the premium in a timely manner.
  — The employee becomes covered under another health plan that contains no limitation or exclusion as to a preexisting condition, or if there is a preexisting condition clause in the policy and the period excluding coverage has ended.
  — The person covered under the continuation policy becomes eligible for Medicare.
  — In the case of dependents who are continuing as part of the employee's continuation election, the person no longer meets the policy's definition of a dependent.

New Mexico: The state continuation policy is limited and includes the following provisions:

▪ If the employee has employer-based group health insurance and his or her employment is terminated, coverage may be extended for a period of six months.

▪ Death, divorce, or legal separation also triggers up to six months of continued coverage for the insured spouse and dependent.

New York: The New York law authorizing continuation of a group health policy closely parallels the federal COBRA statute. The statute includes the following features:

▪ In case of termination of the employee, group health coverage insuring this individual and his or her dependents may be extended for a period of 18 months.

▪ The election to continue must be exercised by the employee within 60 days following the termination or the date he or she was sent notification of continuation by the group policyholder, whichever is later.

- Continuation does not apply to an employee who is eligible for another group policy, provided that it does not contain a preexisting condition limitation.
- Continuation does not apply to an employee eligible for Medicare.
- If the employee is determined to have been disabled under SSDI standards at any time during the first 60 days of continuation of coverage, the coverage may be extended to a period of 29 months.

North Carolina: The North Carolina law provides a COBRA-like policy for employees experiencing termination of employment. The legislation includes the following features:

- If an employee is insured through an employer-sponsored health policy and is terminated from work, he or she will be able to continue coverage for himself, and for eligible spouses and other dependents, for a period of 18 months.
- The premium for the continuation policy is to be no more than the group rate.

North Dakota: Under state law, continuation of an employee's group coverage includes the following features:

- The employee must have been insured for a period of at least three continuous months, ending with the termination.
- Continuation is not available to those employees or dependents who are covered under Medicare.
- If an employee is insured through an employer-sponsored health policy and is terminated from work, he or she will be able to continue coverage for himself and an eligible spouse and other dependents for up to 39 weeks.
- When continuation is due to the termination of employment, the premium charged on a continuation policy may not be more than that charged for the group coverage. However, when continuation is triggered by divorce, the premium may be as high as 102 percent of the group rate.

Ohio: State law provides a program that continues health coverage for an individual insured in a group health plan sponsored by an employer regardless of whether it is subject to COBRA. The legislation includes the following features:

- The employee must be covered under the group policy for three months immediately preceding the termination of his or her employment.
- Continuation does not extend to individuals who are covered under Medicare.
- The term of the continuation policy is six months.

■ Spouses and dependents of reservists called to active duty may extend coverage for up to 36 months if the reservist dies.

Oklahoma: The state continuation policy is limited. It covers the following:

■ If an individual has group health coverage through his or her employer and the insurance is terminated, the employee and dependents will remain insured for a period of at least 30 days following the termination.

Oregon: Oregon's continuation policy legislation covers the following features:

■ If an individual (certificate holder) has group health coverage through his or her employer and the employment has terminated, the employee and dependents may remain insured for six months.
■ The extension commences on the date of termination.
■ Coverage will cease if the certificate holder becomes eligible for Medicare.

Rhode Island: Under state law, the plan will continue for a period of 18 months if the employer provides group health insurance to an employee whose coverage is then terminated because of involuntary layoff, death, the workplace ceasing to exist, or permanent reduction in the size of the workforce. Other features of the statute include the following:

■ The extension covers both the employee and eligible dependents and spouse.
■ The cost of insurance may not exceed the premium charged for the group coverage.

South Carolina: South Carolina's continuation policy legislation includes the following:

■ If an individual has group health coverage through employment and the policy is terminated for any reason other than nonpayment of the premium, the insured is entitled to continue coverage for six months, plus any fraction of a month remaining.
■ The employee must be insured under the policy for at least six months immediately preceding termination.
■ The employer is required to inform the employee of the right to continue coverage following termination of the policy. Notification will occur at the time of termination.
■ The premium charged for the extended coverage may not exceed the group rate.

South Dakota: The state has legislation similar to COBRA and includes the following features:

■ The statute applies only to companies with fewer than 20 employees.

■ Coverage will continue for a term of 18 months.

■ Continuation is available only to the employee who had coverage under the group policy during the entire six-month period prior to the termination.

Tennessee: An employee who was covered under a fully insured group plan for three months or more and lost that coverage may be eligible for up to three months of continued coverage under the same group plan. In addition, a spouse or dependent who lost coverage because of the death of a spouse or divorce may be eligible for up to 15 months of continued coverage. Potential beneficiaries should ask their former employer or the Tennessee Department of Commerce and Insurance if this applies to them.

Texas: Under state law, continuation of the group health coverage includes the following features:

■ An employee's termination of insurance triggers up to six months of continued coverage, provided that the employee had been covered for at least three months immediately preceding termination.

■ Death, divorce, or legal separation triggers up to three years of coverage continuation for the employee's spouse and dependent, provided that they were covered continuously for at least one year before the qualifying event.

■ The premium for continuation coverage may not exceed 102 percent of the group rate.

Utah: The state continuation policy is limited. It includes the following features:

■ An employee's termination of group insurance triggers up to six months of continued coverage, provided that the insured group is not subject to COBRA and the termination is not due to gross misconduct.

■ The new coverage will terminate prior to the completion of the six-month term if one of the following occurs:

— The terminated insured establishes residency outside the state of Utah.

— There is failure to make timely payment of the premium.

— Violation of a material condition of the policy occurs or the employer's coverage is terminated.

— The employer replaces the insurance with a similar group policy coverage.

Vermont: The state has a statute similar to COBRA, but it is not as broad. The legislation includes the following benefits and limitations:

■ An individual who has been insured under an employer-based group health policy and has been continuously covered for a period of three months immediately preceding termination is entitled to up to six months of coverage.

■ The right of continuation does not extend to individuals eligible for another group plan or Medicare.

■ For insured groups not subject to COBRA, death of an employee triggers up to six months of continuation coverage for spouses and dependents.

Virginia: Virginia has a limited COBRA-like statute. The legislation includes the following benefits and limitations:

■ Termination of employment triggers up to 90 days of continued coverage, provided that the insured was covered continuously for at least three months immediately preceding termination.

■ Continuation does not apply to individuals who are eligible for other group coverage or Medicare.

■ The premium for a continuation policy may not exceed the group rate.

Washington: For insured groups, Washington has a continuation statute that includes the following features:

■ The law is not based on coverage through employment. Instead, it requires insurers that provide group health coverage to offer the policyholder the option to include continuation coverage for any person who becomes ineligible for any reason.

■ The premium charged is agreed to by the policyholder and the insurer.

■ The option provided by law requires the policyholder and the insurer to negotiate the terms triggering continuation of coverage.

West Virginia: For insured groups not subject to COBRA, West Virginia has a continuation statute that includes the following features:

■ Coverage will be up to 18 months when an employee who is insured under an employer-sponsored group policy is involuntarily terminated.

■ The continuation applies to all individuals insured by such group coverage.

Wisconsin: For insured groups not subject to COBRA, Wisconsin has a continuation statute that either parallels or is more liberal than the federal statute. The more important features include the following:

■ Continuation extends for a term of 18 months when an employee who is insured under an employer-sponsored group policy is terminated.

■ Notice of the option to continue coverage must be sent within 5 days (not 44 days, as permitted by COBRA) to the insured employee, dependents, or qualified beneficiaries if the loss of coverage is due to termination of employment, death, or total disability.

■ The premium may not exceed the group rate.

■ Continuation of coverage ceases if one of the following occurs:

— The terminated insured establishes residency outside the state of Wisconsin.

— The terminated insured fails to make timely payment of the premium.

— The terminated insured becomes eligible for similar coverage.

Wyoming: For insured groups not subject to the federal statute of COBRA, the state of Wyoming offers the following options:

■ Continuation of COBRA for a fully insured group health plan, or a state or local government plan, with 2 to 19 employees

■ Coverage of up to 12 months when the employee's job ends

12

TICKET TO WORK AND WORK INCENTIVES

On December 17, 1999, President Clinton signed into law the Ticket to Work and Work Incentives Improvement Act (TWWIIA). TWWIIA was enacted to make it easier for individuals with disabilities to receive vocational rehabilitation and employment support, and for them to retain Medicare benefits longer when returning to work. It also removed limits on Medicaid buy-in options for workers with disabilities. The act began being phased in over a four-year period beginning in 2000.

In his comments at the time of passage, President Clinton noted that it was the fear of losing health insurance that kept people with disabilities from seeking employment. This dilemma placed people with disabilities who were receiving Social Security and wanted to work in a "double bind," since keeping health benefits required staying out of the workforce and on Social Security. According to President Clinton, this paradox "defies common sense and economic logic. This is about more than jobs and paychecks. It is fundamentally about the dignity of each human being . . . [in] recognizing that work is at the heart of the American dream." Fear of losing insurance should not keep people from seeking employment.

■ MEDICARE

TWWIIA extends to 8.5 years the premium-free Medicare Part A benefits for people on SSD who return to work. Payment for Part B coverage would continue to be the established annual premium. The legislation also bars the SSA from medically reviewing a beneficiary solely because of his or her work activity.

In addition, the act requires that if the recipient is disabled, entitled to Medicare Part A benefits, and becomes covered under a group health plan through employment (provided that the employer has 20 or more employees), the premiums and benefits for any Medigap plan covering the insured may be suspended at his or her request. If the insured loses the employer coverage after receiving such group insurance and suspending Medigap, the Medigap policy must restore benefits. (However, the renewal of coverage becomes effective only if the individual provides notice of the loss within 90 days of such event.)

■ MEDICAID

The TWWIIA also allows states to provide Medicaid coverage to eligible workers with disabilities. Medicaid options for the states include the following:

■ Make Medicaid available to individuals between the ages of 16 and 64 who, because of income earned from work, are ineligible to receive Supplemental Security Income (SSI); and

■ Extend Medicaid to employed persons with disabilities whose medical condition has improved, but who have continued to have a "severe medically determinable impairment" as defined by the federal Health and Human Services Regulations.

The decision to make these changes to Medicaid is determined by each state. The status of a state's legislation pursuant to this act can be provided by its Department of Insurance. Each state determines its own income cap for participation, and may charge individuals a portion of premium costs on a sliding scale.

Persons in states exercising these options who previously would not have qualified for Medicaid are now permitted to buy into Medicaid coverage by paying premiums and other cost-sharing charges on a sliding-fee scale based on income.

13

COMPREHENSIVE STATE HEALTH INSURANCE FOR HIGH-RISK INDIVIDUALS[1]

High-risk pools have been created by 33 states to provide an insurance option to those who are considered medically uninsurable or high risk. These programs offer an insurance alternative to individuals who have been denied health insurance coverage due to a serious health condition, or whose insurance premiums have escalated beyond those charged in the high-risk pool.

Eligibility for these programs varies from state to state. For several states, individuals are qualified if they meet the standards of federal eligibility. Federal eligibility criteria are as follows:

- Is a current resident of the state
- Has had continuous creditable coverage of 18 months or more, at least the last day of which was under a group health plan or government plan
- Is not eligible for coverage under a group health plan, Medicare, or Medicaid
- Has not had a break in coverage for 63 or more days from the time the previous insurance was terminated
- Has exhausted all COBRA or similar state program benefits

---

[1]The information in this chapter was collected from several sources, including: *Comprehensive Health Insurance for High-Risk Individuals: A State-by-State Analysis; Communicating for Agriculture: 1999; State Coverage Initiatives: An Initiative of the Robert Wood Johnson Foundation, 2006;* state offices for high-risk insurance pools; and the Georgetown University website www.healthinsuranceinfo.net.

■ ALABAMA

Organization Administering Insurance and Contact

Organization: Alabama Health Insurance

State contact:

Alabama Health Insurance Plan (AHIP)
c/o State Employees Insurance Board
P.O. Box 304900
Montgomery, AL 36130-4900
877-619-2447

Eligibility Criteria and Premium Cap

The applicant

■ Must be an Alabama resident;

■ Must be eligible for portability under the Health Insurance and Portability and Accountability Act (HIPAA);

■ Must have had at least 18 months of continuous previous coverage;

■ Must have exhausted COBRA coverage if eligible;

■ Must have not had a break in coverage of 63 or more days from the time the previous insurance was terminated;

■ Must have been last insured under either a group health plan, a government plan, or a church plan; and

■ Must not have had previous coverage terminated because of fraud or failure to pay premiums.

Premium cap: The cap is fixed at 200 percent of the standard market rate for comparable health insurance.

Waiting Period for Preexisting Conditions and Waiver of Waiting Period

■ *Waiting period for preexisting conditions:* None

■ *Waiver of waiting period:* None

Coverage

Two companies provide high-risk insurance in Alabama: Blue Cross/Blue Shield and United Health Care.

Blue Cross administers a traditional indemnity plan that offers annual deductibles of $1,000 (Plan C) and $2,500 (Plan D). Both the C and D plans limit the annual out-of-pocket costs to $1,500 per person plus any hospital stay deductible amount. Once the deductible amounts are reached, both plans pay 80 percent of the usual, reasonable, and customary charges of the item covered. After the out-of-pocket limit is reached, the plans pay 100 percent of that charge.

United Health Care makes available an HMO plan with no deductible except for prescription drugs. Features of this plan include

- Inpatient hospitalization (co-pay)
- Outpatient care/doctor visits (co-pay)
- Prescription drug coverage (with a maximum annual benefit, per insured, of $1,500)
- Ambulance (co-pay)
- Skilled nursing care (x limited days)
- Home health visits (a limitation on visits applies)
- Durable medical equipment (an annual limit applies)
- Physical therapy (co-pay and annual limit on visits)

Lifetime benefit: $1,000,000

■ ALASKA

Organization Administering Insurance and Contact

Organization: Alaska Comprehensive Health Insurance (ACHI)

State contact:

Alaska Comprehensive Health Insurance
2015 16th Street
Great Bend, KS 67530
888-290-0616

Eligibility Criteria and Premium Cap

Under the state high-risk rules, a person is eligible for coverage if

■ The applicant has been a resident of the state for a period of at least 12 months;

■ The applicant is not eligible to have been covered under the state's small employer health insurance plan (2 to 50 employees);

■ The applicant is not insured under another health plan, including a government health plan (i.e., Medicare) or a group health plan; and

■ At least one of the following has occurred:

– Applicant has received notice of rejection for health insurance from at least one health insurer.

– Applicant has one of the listed conditions qualifying for coverage.

– Applicant has received restrictive riders that substantially reduce coverage.

Under the federal rules, a person is also eligible for coverage if

■ He or she is domiciled in the state of Alaska;

■ He or she has had 18 months of prior health coverage without a break for 90 days in coverage;

■ The most recent health insurance was structured as a group plan;

■ The most recent coverage was not terminated because of fraud or nonpayment of a premium;

■ He or she is not eligible for Medicare, Medicaid, Indian Health Services, or other group health insurance coverage; and

■ He or she is not covered under another health insurance plan.

Premium cap: The cap is fixed at 200 percent of the standard rate for comparable coverage.

Waiting Period for Preexisting Conditions and Waiver of Waiting Period

■ *Waiting period for preexisting conditions:* If the individual is not federally eligible, coverage will not be extended for expenses incurred during the first six months following the effective date of coverage for any condition if (a) the condition manifested itself within the three-month period immediately preceding the effective date of coverage; or (b) medical advice, care, or treatment was recommended or received for such condition within the first three-month period immediately preceding the effective date of coverage.

■ *Waiver of waiting period:* If the insured's previous plan was involuntarily terminated, the time covered under the earlier policy will be credited toward the preexisting condition period of the new state policy, provided that the person applies for the new plan within 31 days after termination of the previous contract.

Coverage

The policies offered include

1. A major medical PPO plan with per-individual deductibles at $1,000, $1,500, $2,500, $5,000, and $10,000. For the $1,000 deductible, the insured is subject to a $2,500 out-of-pocket expense limitation; for the $1,500 deductible, a $3,000 out-of-pocket limit; for the $2,500 deductible, a $5,000 out-of-pocket limit; for the $5,000 deductible, a $10,000 out-of-pocket limit; and for the $10,000 deductible, a $15,000 out-of-pocket limit. The annual deductible is the amount that the insured must pay each calendar year for eligible expenses before the plan pays benefits, and the out-of-pocket expense limitation is the maximum amount to be paid any calendar year. Once the deductible is paid, the insurer is responsible for 80 percent of the usual and customary charge for in-network expenses and 60 percent of such charge for out-of-network costs. Once the out-of-pocket amounts are paid, the insurance picks up 100 percent of the provider charges regardless of whether it is in-network or out-of network.

2. A major medical indemnity plan with a single deductible of $1,000 and an out-of-pocket limitation of $2,500.

3. A Medicare carve-out plan, which is the same as the indemnity plan except for lower premiums for the insured and the coordination of benefits between ACHI and Medicare.

The benefits offered under the Alaska plan include the following:

■ Inpatient hospital expense
■ Outpatient care/doctor visits
■ Prescription drug coverage, except for Medicare-eligible individuals
■ Ambulance
■ Skilled nursing care (limited days per year)

- Home health care (limited visits per year)
- Durable medical equipment
- Physical therapy

Lifetime benefit: $1,000,000

■ ARKANSAS

Organization Administering Insurance and Contact

Organization:Arkansas Comprehensive Health Insurance Pool (CHIP)
State contact:

Arkansas Comprehensive Health Insurance Pool
P.O. Box 419
Little Rock, AR 72203
501-370-2659
800-285-6477

Eligibility Criteria and Premium Cap

Individuals qualify if they are federally eligible. An individual who is not federally eligible will also qualify if he or she meets the following criteria:

- Is a resident of Arkansas for a period of at least 30 days; and
- Was rejected by an insurer for substantially similar coverage because of a preexisting medical condition; or
- Was offered coverage in excess of the premium for high-risk insurance; or
- Has one of the listed conditions qualifying the applicant for coverage; and
- Is not eligible for or already has similar coverage from another health plan.

Premium cap: The premium is capped at 150 percent of the standard rate for comparable coverage.

Waiting Period for Preexisting Conditions and Waiver of Waiting Period

- *Waiting period for preexisting conditions:* If the individual is not federally eligible, coverage will not be extended to expenses incurred during the first six months following the effective date of coverage for any condition if (a) the condition manifested itself within the six-month period immediately preceding the effective date of coverage, or (b) medical advice, care, or treatment was recommended or received as to such condition within the first six-month period immediately preceding the effective date of coverage.

■ *Waiver of waiting period:* If the applicant is either federally eligible or his or her previous plan was involuntarily terminated, the time covered under the earlier policy will be credited toward the preexisting condition period of the new state policy provided that the person applies for the new plan within 31 days after termination of the previous contract.

Coverage

The Arkansas plan is structured as a PPO with three deductible amounts offered: $1,000, $5,000, and $10,000. Once the deductible is met, there will be an 80/20 payment made for in-network expenses and a 60/40 payment for out-of-network expenses until the covered expenses reach $5,000 for a $1,000 deductible, $25,000 for a $5,000 deductible, or $50,000 for a $10,000 deductible. All covered expenses incurred thereafter during the plan year are paid at 100 percent.

The benefits offered in the Arkansas plan include the following:

■ Hospital services

■ Professional services for the diagnosis or treatment of injuries or conditions, other than dental, that are rendered by a physician or by others at his or her direction

■ Drugs requiring a physician's prescription

■ Services of a licensed skilled nursing facility for individuals ineligible for Medicare, for not more than 180 calendar days during a policy year, provided that the services are of the type that would qualify as reimbursable services under Medicare

■ Services of a home health agency

■ Rental or purchase, as appropriate, of durable medical equipment

■ Services of a physical therapist and diagnostic X-rays and laboratory tests

Lifetime benefit: $1,000,000

■ CALIFORNIA

Organization Administering Insurance and Contact

Organization: California Major Medical Insurance
State contact:
    Managed Risk Medical Insurance Program (MRMIP)
    P.O. Box 2769
    Sacramento, CA 95812-2769
    800-289-6574

Eligibility Criteria and Premium Cap

In order to be eligible for coverage, the insured must meet the following criteria:

▪ Be a resident of the State of California

▪ Not be eligible for Part A and Part B of Medicare

▪ Not be eligible for COBRA or Cal-COBRA benefits

▪ Be able to demonstrate an inability to secure adequate coverage within the previous 12 months due to being

 – Denied insurance coverage;

 – Involuntarily terminated for reasons other than nonpayment of premium or fraud;

 – Requested to pay premium in excess of the program subscriber rate; or

 – A member of a group that has been denied coverage.

Premium cap: The premium cap tends to be 25 to 37.5 percent above the standard market rate for comparable health insurance.

Waiting Period for Preexisting Conditions, Waiver of Waiting Period, and Wait List for Program

▪ Waiting period for preexisting conditions: For individuals enrolling in the pool's PPO plan, coverage is excluded during a 90-day period following the effective date of coverage for any condition for which medical advice, care, or treatment was recommended or received during the six months immediately preceding enrollment.

▪ For individuals enrolling in the pool's HMO plan, there is a post-enrollment waiting period of 90 days. Subscribers will not be eligible for benefits during this period.

▪ Waiver of waiting period: The waiting period may be waived in part or all if the subscriber

 – Has fulfilled the waiting period under prior coverage and applied within 63 days of loss of coverage

 – Has been on the pool's waiting list for a period of at least six months

 – Has had coverage with an employer that ended because of loss of job, or the employer stopped offering health insurance, or the employer stopped contributing to the health plan, and application was made within 180 days of termination of coverage

- Was insured under a high-risk pool offered in another state within the previous 12 months
■ *Waiting list:* The California program maintains a waiting list for new enrollees. The average wait is four to six months, which is credited toward the waiting period.

Coverage

Under recent legislation California's Managed Risk Medical Insurance Program was changed from a high-risk pool to a "short-term incubator." After three years people enrolled in the pool are granted "guaranteed eligibility" in the individual insurance market if they enroll within 63 days of the MRMIP end date.

Several insurance plans are offered by the Major Risk Medical Insurance Program. Following is a brief description of each plan. All plans offer first-dollar coverage with co-pays.

■ *Blue Cross of California:* The plan is structured as a PPO with no annual deductible. There is prescription drug coverage consisting of pharmacy and mail order service, a limitation in the co-pay for office visits to in-network doctors , and an out-of-pocket maximum for in-network services of $2,500 per insured with a $4,000 maximum per family.

■ *Blue Shield Access + HMO:* The Blue Shield Access + HMO plan provides each subscriber with a personal physician who coordinates all health care needs, including medically necessary X-ray, laboratory, emergency, and hospital services. The charge for physician care within the group is a fixed co-pay for office visits, and the cost of prescriptive drugs is fixed for generic and brand-name medications. The maximum annual amount in co-payments is $2,500 per individual and $4,000 per family.

■ *Kaiser Permanente Northern California Region:* The insurer arranges medical care at its medical facilities. Laboratories, X-ray services, and pharmacies are also located in the facilities. The plan has no deductible, and the out-of-pocket maximum is $2,500 per covered person and $4,000 per family. Physician care requires a small co-pay per office visit, and prescription drugs have co-pays based on generic and brand names.

■ Kaiser Permanente Southern California: The benefits are the same as for the Kaiser Permanente Northern California plan.

Lifetime benefit: $750,000 ($75,000 annual)

■ COLORADO

Organization Administering Insurance and Contact

Organization: CoverColorado

State contact:

425 South Cherry Street
Suite 160
Glendale, CO 80246
877-461-3811

Eligibility Criteria and Premium Cap

■ Applicant must be a U.S. citizen or have legal alien status.

Applicant must be a permanent resident of Colorado for at least six months, must not be delinquent in the payment of Colorado income taxes, and must meet one of the following conditions after having applied for health coverage:

- The application was rejected because of a medical condition;
- The application was accepted, but the premium was higher than the premium under the state's high-risk plan;
- The application was accepted, but treatment of preexisting health conditions would be permanently excluded; or
- The applicant has one of the medical conditions listed in the insurance application form.

Premium cap: The cap is fixed at 150 percent of the standard rate for comparable coverage.

Waiting Period for Preexisting Conditions and Waiver of Waiting Period

■ *Waiting period for preexisting conditions:* Coverage is excluded during the six-month period following the effective date of coverage for any condition that was recommended or received during the six-month period immediately preceding enrollment medical advice, care, or treatment.

■ *Waiver of waiting period:* A full or partial waiver of the waiting period is offered to those individuals who had qualifying previous coverage that was terminated no more than 90 days prior to CoverColorado coverage.

Coverage

Colorado offers a statewide major medical plan with five deductible levels to choose from, using PacifiCare PPO network and an HSA plan. The plan includes the following features:

- *Deductible:* The deductible amounts offered for the PPO range from $1,000 to over $10,000.
- *Outpatient care/doctor visits:* The PPO coverage for an in-network provider is 80/20. The cost for an out-of-network provider will average 50 percent.
- *Inpatient hospital expense:* The PPO has the same co-insurance as provided for doctor visits.
- *Prescription drug coverage:* Prescription drug coverage ranges, depending on the plan selected.
- *Ambulance.*
- *Home health care:* A limitation on visits per year applies.
- *Physical therapy:* Pre-certification is required for more than six visits.
- *Annual participant out-of-pocket maximum:* The out-of-pocket maximum will vary according to plan deductible that is selected.

Lifetime benefit: $1,000,000

■ CONNECTICUT

Organization Administering Insurance and Contact

Organization: Connecticut Health Reinsurance Association (CHRA)
State contact:
Connecticut Health Reinsurance Association
100 Great Meadow Road, Suite 704
Weathersfield, CT 06109
800-842-0004

Eligibility Criteria and Premium Cap

The individual applying for coverage must be a state resident between the ages of 19 and 65. Unlike a number of state plans, Connecticut requires the applicant to be rejected by a health insurer prior to applying for its plan. Individuals also qualify if they are federally eligible.

Premium cap: Premiums may not be greater than 150–200 percent of the standard charge for comparable coverage.

Waiting Period for Preexisting Conditions and Waiver of Waiting Period

▪ *Individual policy:* If the insured was covered under an individual policy and has an existing medical condition, coverage is excluded for the first 12 months following the effective date of the CHRA policy. Coverage is also excluded during this 12-month period for the individual policyholder as to any condition for which treatment was received during the six-month period immediately preceding enrollment.

▪ *Group insurance:* If the insured was covered under a qualifying group plan

    – For more than 12 months, there are no preexisting coverage limitations.

    – For less than 12 months, coverage for a preexisting condition will be provided under the CHRA policy when the insured has been covered for a total of 12 months between the prior group policy and the CHRA policy.

▪ *Federal eligibility:* The waiting period is waived if the insured is federally eligible.

Coverage

Connecticut offers three plans for enrollment. There are two individual plans, which are PPOs administered by the Special Health Care plan and the United HealthCare PPO plan. There are also conversion plans and portability plans, including a HealthNet HMO option.

The PPO plan also has a $2,500 per-individual maximum out-of-pocket cost when the insured uses an in-network provider. The family out-of-pocket maximum is $5,000. Services in the PPO tend to be 80/20 after the deductible for in-network providers and 60/40 after the deductible for out-of-network providers.

Services covered include

▪ Physician services
▪ Office visits
▪ Surgery
▪ Hospital services

■ Emergency room

■ X-rays and lab exams

■ Outpatient drugs

The HMO plan has a maximum out-of-pocket cost for in-network providers of $2,500 per individual and $5,000 per family. There is no annual deductible (except for hospital and skilled nursing services) and small co-payments for physician visits, home health care, and outpatient prescription drugs.

Lifetime benefit: $1,000,000

■ FLORIDA

Organization Administering Insurance and Contact

Organization:Florida Comprehensive Health Association (FCHA)

State contact:

FCHA
1210 East Park Avenue
Tallahassee, FL 32301
850-309-1200

Note: The Florida Legislature closed new enrollment in the plan effective June 30, 1991.

Approximately 500 individuals remain in the program as of 2006. Premium caps vary between 200 and 250 percent.

■ IDAHO

Organization Administering Insurance and Contact

■ Organization: High Risk Reinsurance Pool Plans

■ State contact:

Idaho Department of Insurance
700 West State Street, 3rd floor
Boise, ID 83720-0043
208-334-4250
800-721-3272

Eligibility Criteria and Premium Cap

The applicant

- Must be an Idaho resident or dependent on an Idaho resident, and
- Must be federally eligible under HIPAA, or
- Must have been declined coverage due to health status or claims experience, or
- Must have been offered coverage similar to the HRP plan but at a higher premium rate

Premium cap: All carriers must charge the same premium rates set for the five plans by the HRP Board of Directors.

Waiting Period for Preexisting Conditions and Waiver of Waiting Period

- *Waiting period for preexisting conditions:* An HRP plan may exclude benefits for a preexisting condition for 12 months after the effective date of coverage. However, if the individual is covered under a group or individual plan within 63 days before applying, credit will be given for the time insured toward this 12-month exclusion.
- *Waiver of waiting period:* No preexisting exclusion may be applied under the HRP plan to those who are "federally eligible" if the individual applies within 63 days of termination of prior creditable coverage.

Coverage

There are five HRP plans: Basic, Standard, Catastrophic A, Catastrophic B, and HSA Compatible. An applicant has the right to choose any one of the five plans. Deductibles range from $500 for the basic plan to $5,000 for the Catastrophic B plan. Co-insurance, out-of-pocket expense maximums, and coverage for drugs vary among the plans. Benefit areas such as the following also vary by plan selected:

- Preventive services
- Organ transplant
- Skilled nursing facility
- Rehabilitation therapy
- Home health care
- Durable medical equipment

Lifetime benefit: $1,000,000 for the Catastrophic A and B plans; $500,000 for the other plans

■ ILLINOIS

Organization Administering Insurance and Contact

Organization: Illinois Comprehensive Health Insurance (ICHI)

State contact:

Illinois Comprehensive Health Insurance
320 West Washington Street, Suite 300
Springfield, IL 62701
866-851-2751

Eligibility Criteria and Premium Cap

Three types of plans are offered in the Illinois high-risk pool:

■ Plan 2 is available only to individuals under the age of 65 who are enrolled in Parts A and B of Medicare due to a disability or have end-stage renal disease.

■ Plan 3 is a PPO plan, available only to eligible persons who qualify for CHIP and are not eligible for Medicare. To attain maximum benefits under this plan, a designated PPO provider must be used.

■ Plan 5 is a PPO plan available only to federally eligible individuals. There is no preexisting condition limitation in this plan.

Federal eligibility allows individuals to avoid a preexisting condition waiting period, even if they have changed insurance plans. An individuals who is not federally eligible and is applying for Plan 2 or 3 must

■ Be a U.S. citizen or permanent resident alien;

■ Be a resident of Illinois for at least 180 days;

■ Have applied to an insurance company within the last nine months and received a rejection or refusal to issue the insurance for health reasons by one insurer;

■ Have received a refusal to issue or renew substantially similar individual health coverage at a rate exceeding the amount charged for the ICHIP plan; or

■ Have been diagnosed with one of 31 presumptive medical conditions.

Premium cap: The premium is based on the insured's age, sex, and county of residence. Premiums are usually set at 135 percent of the average cost for comparable service.

Waiting Period for Preexisting Conditions and Waiver of Waiting Period

■ *Waiting period for preexisting conditions:* For those individuals who are not federally eligible, coverage is excluded during the six-month period following the effective date of coverage for any condition for which medical advice, care, or treatment was recommended or received during the six-month period immediately preceding the enrollment.

■ *Waiver of waiting period:* A waiver is granted if the individual's insurance immediately preceding the ICHI policy was involuntarily terminated; if the individual is ineligible for any continuation or conversion rights; if application for ICHI and waiver is made within 90 days following termination; and with payment of an additional 10 percent increase in the regular premium for the life of the policy or 60 months, whichever is less.

Coverage

Two of the plans offered by Illinois are structured as PPOs and one as a major medical plan. Individual deductibles and out-of-pocket expenses vary with the plan. Each of the benefit plans offers deductible options of $500, $1,000, $1,500, $2,500, and $5,000.

The benefits provided under the Illinois plans include

■ Daily room and board and other hospital services

■ Professional medical services

■ Purchase or rental of durable medical equipment

■ Skilled nursing care benefits limited to 120 days in a skilled nursing facility each calendar year

■ Physical therapy

■ Diagnostic services

Lifetime benefit: $1,000,000

■ INDIANA

Organization Administering Insurance and Contact

Organization: Indiana Comprehensive Health Insurance Association (ICHIA)
State contact
Indiana Comprehensive Health Insurance Association
P.O. Box 33730
Indianapolis, IN 46203
800-552-7921
317-614-2133

Eligibility Criteria and Premium Cap

■ Participants must be a resident of the state for at least 12 months immediately preceding the application for insurance unless they are federally eligible, or

■ They cannot be eligible for a group health insurance plan, and they have received or qualified for one of the following:

- A notice of rejection for substantially similar insurance, or

- A notice for health insurance coverage exceeding the premium rate for coverage under ICHIA.

An individual will always qualify if he or she is federally eligible.

Premium cap: The figure is capped at 150 percent of the standard rate for comparable coverage.

Waiting Period for Preexisting Conditions and Waiver of Waiting Period

■ *Waiting period for preexisting conditions:* Coverage is excluded during the three-month period following the effective date of coverage for any condition for which medical advice, care, or treatment was recommended or received during the three-month period immediately preceding enrollment.

■ *Waiver of waiting period:* The waiting period is waived if the participant was covered for health insurance and lost coverage within six months prior to application for ICHIA insurance. Federal eligibility also allows individuals to avoid a preexisting condition waiting period.

Coverage

Indiana offers four plans that include a PPO benefit. In-network charges are usually covered at an 80/20 ratio and out-of-network at 60/40. Each plan has its own deductible, co-insurance, and benefit costs. For example,

■ Plan 1 has a $500 deductible. The out-of-pocket limit for an individual is $1,500.

■ Plan 2 has a $1,000 deductible. The out-of-pocket limit for an individual is $3,000.

■ Plan 3 has a $1,500 deductible and an out-of pocket limit of $5,000.

The following are covered under the three plans:

■ Inpatient and outpatient hospital services

■ Skilled nursing care service

■ Noncustodial home health care services

■ Surgical and transplant services

■ Prescription drug coverage through Anthem Prescription Drug Network

Lifetime benefit: No maximum lifetime benefit

■ IOWA

Organization Administering Insurance and Contact

Organization: Health Insurance Plan of Iowa (HIPIOWA)

State contact:

Health Insurance Plan of Iowa
P.O. Box 1090
Great Bend, KS 67530
877-793-6880

Eligibility Criteria and Premium Cap

The participant must be a resident of Iowa for at least 60 days and meet one of the following eligibility criteria:

■ Notice of rejection for substantially similar health insurance dated within the last nine months

■ Notice of benefit reduction or specific condition exclusion

■ Notice of premium increase for similar coverage that exceeds the ICHA policy rate

Coverage is also available to people who have resided in Iowa for 60 days and have been diagnosed with a condition listed on the plan brochure. In this instance, the above items do not have to be satisfied.

An individual may also qualify if he or she is federally eligible.

Premium cap: The figure is capped at 150 percent of the standard rate for health insurance in the state.

Waiting Period for Preexisting Conditions and Waiver of Waiting Period

■ *Waiting period:* Coverage is excluded during the six-month period following the effective date of coverage for any condition for which medical advice, care, or treatment was recommended or received during the six-month period immediately preceding enrollment.

■ *Waiver of waiting period:* The waiting period is waived if (a) the preexisting condition factor has been satisfied with the previous carrier, (b) the previous coverage was involuntarily terminated, (c) there was not a conversion policy offered with similar coverage and lower rates, and (d) application for the high-risk insurance is received within 63 days from the date the previous policy was canceled. A waiver is also granted if the applicant is federally eligible as of the date he or she seeks coverage.

Coverage

The following types of plans are offered:

■ *Plan Option A (A Medicare carve-out)*
  – Annual deductible: $1,000 per insured
  – Out-of-pocket limit including deductible: $2,500 for in-network and $5,000 for out-of-network
  – Co-insurance: 80 percent for in-network and 60 percent for out-of-network

■ *Plan Option B*
  – Annual deductible: $1,000 per insured
  – Out-of-pocket limit including deductible: $2,500 for in-network and $5,000 for out-of-network
  – Co-insurance: 80 percent for in-network and 60 percent for out-of-network

■ *Plan Option C*
  – Annual deductible: $1,500 per insured
  – Out-of-pocket limit including deductible: $3,000 for in-network and $6,000 for out-of-network
  – Co-insurance: 80 percent for in-network and 60 percent for out-of-network

■ *Plan Option D*
  – Annual deductible: $2,500 per insured
  – Out-of-pocket limit including deductible: $5,000 for in-network and 10,000 for out-of-network
  – Co-insurance: 80 percent for in-network and 60 percent for out-of-network

The Iowa plan includes the following services:

- Inpatient care/hospital
- Outpatient care/doctor visits
- Prescription drug coverage
- Skilled nursing care
- Home health visits
- Durable medical equipment
- Physical therapy

Lifetime benefit: $3,000,000

▪ KANSAS

Organization Administering Insurance and Contact

Organization: Kansas Health Insurance Association (KHIA)
State contact:
Kansas Health Insurance Association
P.O. Box 1090
Great Bend, KS 67530
800-362-9290

Eligibility Criteria and Premium Cap

A participant must be eligible because of a medical condition or meet the standards prescribed for federal eligibility.
To qualify for medical condition eligibility,

- An applicant must have been a resident of Kansas for six months.
- He or she must be ineligible for coverage under federal and state programs, including Medicaid or a group health plan.
- He or she must have been offered coverage at a rate higher than the KHIA plan, or
- He or she must have been refused health coverage by two carriers because of a health condition, or
- He or she must have been involuntarily terminated from a health insurance plan for any reason other than nonpayment of premium.

Premium cap: The premium is to be no higher than 125 percent of the market rate for comparable coverage.

Waiting Period for Preexisting Conditions and Waiver of Waiting Period

■ *Waiting period for preexisting conditions:* Benefits are not covered for any preexisting condition for the first 90 days following the effective date of coverage. A preexisting condition is defined as any condition for which medical advice, care, or treatment was recommended or received from a medical practitioner during the six-month period proceeding the effective date of coverage.

■ *Waiver of waiting period:* If the insured is covered under another policy that provides hospital, medical, or surgical benefits, and coverage under that policy terminates less than 31 days prior to coverage beginning under the new plan, the 90-day period will be waived to the extent that the preexisting condition limitation period was satisfied under the previous policy. A preexisting condition waiting period does not apply to an insured who is federally eligible.

Coverage

KHIA offers six PPO plans with six deductibles, ranging from $500 to $7,500. Plan D meets the requirements for a Health Savings Account (HSA). The co-insurance is 70/30 for in-network expenses after the deductible is met, adjusted to 90/10 after payment of the annual maximum. Out-of-network payments are limited to 50 percent of the charge. Coverage under the plan includes:

■ Inpatient hospital expenses
■ Outpatient care/doctor visits
■ Prescription drug coverage
■ Durable medical equipment (subject to deductible and co-insurance levels)
■ Physical therapy (subject to deductible and co-insurance levels)
■ Skilled nursing care (subject to deductible and co-insurance levels)
■ Home health visits (subject to deductible and co-insurance levels)

Lifetime benefit: $1,000,000

■ KENTUCKY

Organization Administering Insurance and Contact

Organization: Kentucky Access
State contact:
    Kentucky Access
    P.O. Box 33707
    Indianapolis, IN 46203-0707
    866-405-6145

Eligibility Criteria and Premium Cap

To be eligible, an applicant

■ Must have been a resident of Kentucky for 12 months;

■ Must be ineligible for insurance providing comparable coverage; and

■ Must meet one of the following eligibility categories:

- Has been refused health coverage by two carriers because of health condition;

- Has been diagnosed with a medical condition that automatically qualifies him or her for Kentucky Access; or

- Has received notice of premium increase for similar coverage that exceeds the Kentucky Access policy rate.

An individual may also qualify if he or she is federally eligible.

Premium cap: The premium cap is 175 percent.

Waiting Period for Preexisting Conditions and Waiver of Waiting Period

■ *Waiting period for preexisting conditions:* Benefits are not covered for any preexisting condition for 12 months following the effective date of coverage. A preexisting condition is defined as any condition for which medical advice, care, or treatment was recommended or received from a medical practitioner during the six-month period proceeding the effective date of coverage.

■ *Waiver of waiting period:* A waiting period of 12 consecutive months will be reduced by the number of days the qualifying previous plan was in effect. A reduction in this waiting period is allowed only if there is no break in coverage greater than 62 days between two plans.

Coverage

Two PPO plans (Premier Access and Preferred Access) and a fee-for-service plan (Traditional Access) are offered by the Kentucky Access program.

The indemnity plan provides a $400 individual and an $800 family deductible. The individual deductible is subject to a maximum out-of-pocket payment of $1,500 after the deductible has been met. The family deductible is subject to a maximum out-of-pocket payment of $3,000 after the deductible has been met.

The PPOs offer a range of deductibles. In the more expensive of the two plans, the co-insurance ranges from 10 to 20 percent for in-network services and 35 to 40 percent for out-of-network care. In the other PPO, the in-network services range from 20 to 50 percent, and the out-of-network services from 40 to 50 percent.

The coverage under the plan includes

- Inpatient hospital expense
- Outpatient care/doctor visits
- Prescription drug coverage
- Durable medical equipment
- Physical therapy
- Skilled nursing care
- Home health visits

Lifetime benefit: $2,000,000

■ LOUISIANA

Organization Administering Insurance and Contact

Organization: Louisiana Health Insurance Association

State contact:

Louisiana Health Plan (LHP)
P.O. Drawer 83880
Baton Rouge, LA 70884-3880
800-736-0947

Eligibility Criteria and Premium Cap

There are three ways to become eligible for LHP:

- Federal eligibility
- Involuntary loss of coverage where the participant
  - Lost coverage after being insured under major medical continuously
  - Did not have a break in coverage of 63 or more days from the time the previous insurance was terminated

■ Proof of uninsurability meeting the following criteria:

- Louisiana resident for at least six months;
- Had application rejected within one year by two insurance companies; or
- Had received notice of premium increase for similar coverage that is at least twice the LHP rate.

Premium cap: The premium is initially capped at 125 percent of the standard rate for comparable coverage. Thereafter, the premium may not exceed 200 percent of the standard rate.

Waiting Period for Preexisting Conditions and Waiver of Waiting Period

■ *Waiting period for preexisting conditions:* Coverage is excluded during the six-month period following the effective date of coverage for any condition for which medical advice, care, or treatment was recommended or received during the six-month period immediately preceding enrollment.

■ *Waiver of waiting period:* A full or partial waiver of the waiting period is offered to those individuals who had qualifying previous coverage that had been terminated no more than 63 days prior to the LHP coverage. Individuals who are federally eligible are not subject to a waiting period.

Coverage

Louisiana offers four individual PPO plans with deductibles at $1,000 (Plan A), $2,000 (Plan B), $3,500 (Plan C), and $5,000 (Plan D). The co-insurance is generally 75/25 for provider services. The coverage under the plan includes

■ Out-of-pocket maximum: Varies by plan, ranging from $1,500 to $4,500.

■ Inpatient hospital expenses.

■ Outpatient care/doctor visits.

■ Prescription drug coverage: Name-brand drugs are covered at 70 percent, generics at 80 percent, and mail order at 90 percent. There is a $15,000 per calendar year maximum.

■ Skilled nursing care (limited to 120 days per calendar year).

■ Home health visits (limited to 270 days per calendar year).

Lifetime benefit: $500,000; $100,000 annually

■ MARYLAND

Organization Administering Insurance and Contact

Organization: Maryland Health Insurance Plan (MHIP)
State contact:
  Maryland Health Insurance Plan
  509 Progress Drive, Suite 117
  Linthicum, MD 21090
  866-780-7105

Eligibility Criteria and Premium Cap

A participant may be eligible for the Maryland Health Insurance Plan if he or she is a resident of Maryland and

■ Is not eligible for group health coverage, COBRA, the Maryland Medical Assistance or Children's Health Program, Medicare, or any other government-sponsored health insurance program;

■ Has exhausted all available group coverage or moved to Maryland from another state's high-risk pool;

■ Has, or has been offered, health insurance that provides limited or restricted coverage, or that excludes coverage for a specific medical condition or conditions;

■ Has been refused individual health insurance for medical reasons or has a specified medical condition.

Premium cap: Determined by plan benefit options, enrollment coverage options, and age of the oldest individual on the policy.

Waiting Period for Preexisting Conditions and Waiver of Waiting Period

None noted in plan material.

Coverage

In the Maryland Health Insurance Plan, there are four plan options from which to make a choice:

- EPO Network Plan
- PPO plan with $500 medical deductible
- PPO plan with $1,000 medical deductible
- High-deductible health plan (HDP) with $1,200 combined medical and pharmacy deductible

In the EPO Network Plan, participants must choose a primary care provider, and they must use only providers within the plan network except in an emergency. The PPO plans and the HDP allow participants to be seen by providers either in-network or out-of-network. The co-insurance to be paid by the participant will be 20 percent for the former and 40 percent for the latter. Benefits include the following:

- Outpatient services
- Hospital inpatient admissions: medical, surgical, and rehabilitation
- Durable medical equipment
- Home health
- Radiology
- Rehabilitation
- Skilled nursing

Lifetime benefit: $2,000,000

▪ MINNESOTA

Organization Administering Insurance and Contact

Organization: Minnesota Comprehensive Health Association (MCHA)
State contact:
    Minnesota Comprehensive Health Association
    5775 Wayzata Boulevard, Suite 910
    St. Louis Park, MN 55416
    952-593-9609

Eligibility Criteria and Premium Cap

A participant must

- Be a resident of Minnesota for six months and
- Have been refused health coverage,

- Have been offered coverage at a higher-than-standard premium, or
- Have been offered health coverage with a restrictive rider or preexisting condition limitation that reduces coverage within six months of the date of enrollment.

In addition, any resident who has been treated within the last three years for one of the presumptive conditions approved by the Minnesota Department of Commerce is automatically eligible for coverage.

Individuals are also eligible if they meet the standards for federal eligibility.
Premium cap: The cap is 125 percent of the weighted average of rates charged by a majority of the insurers and HMOs offering similar coverage.

Waiting Period for Preexisting Conditions and Waiver of Waiting Period

- *Waiting period for preexisting conditions:* Coverage is excluded during the six-month period following the effective date of coverage for any condition for which medical advice, care, or treatment was recommended or received during the six-month period immediately preceding enrollment.
- *Waiver of waiting period:* A full or partial waiver of the waiting period is offered to those individuals who had qualifying previous coverage that had been terminated no more than 90 days prior to the LHP coverage. Individuals who are federally eligible are not subject to a waiting period.

Coverage

Minnesota offers seven individual plan options with deductibles ranging from $500 to $10,000, as well as two Medicare supplement plans:

- $500 deductible plan option
- $1,000 deductible plan option
- $2,000 deductible plan option
- $5,000 deductible plan option
- $10,000 deductible plan option

Once payment of the deductible is met, coverage is provided at 80 percent of the allowed amount for eligible services received from in-network providers. Payment of the remaining 20 percent of charges is a co-insurance and the responsibility of the insured. Once $3,000 of eligible out-of-pocket expenses have been satisfied in a calendar year (for the $5,000 and $10,000 deductible plans, the deductible amount serves as the out-of-pocket maximum), MCHA pays 100 percent of the allowed amount for eligible services to the end of the calendar year. There is an option to utilize out-of-network providers. However, the benefit and payment percentage will generally be less than stated above. Benefits provided under the plans include the following:

- Hospital services
- Professional services for the diagnosis or treatment of injuries, illnesses, or conditions
- Prescription drug coverage (for coverage under the Medicare policies, limited prescription drugs are included only in the Extended Plan)
- Services of a nursing home for not more than 120 days, provided that the services qualify under Medicare
- Services of a home health agency if the services would qualify under Medicare
- Opinion of a second physician on surgical procedures
- Outpatient doctor visits
- Physical therapy

Lifetime benefit: $2,800,000

■ MISSISSIPPI

Organization Administering Insurance and Contact

> Organization: Mississippi Comprehensive Health Insurance Risk Pool Association (MCHIRP)
>
> State contact:
>> Mississippi Comprehensive Health Insurance Risk Pool Association
>> P.O. Box 13748
>> Jackson, MS 39236
>> 601-899-9967
>> 888-820-9400

Eligibility Criteria and Premium Cap

There are two ways to become eligible. Individuals qualify if they are federally eligible. For individuals who are not federally eligible, the following standards must be met:

- Participants must be a legal resident of the state for six months; and
- Must have an automatically rejectable health condition,
- During the 12 months preceding application, have been rejected by one insurer,
- Have been offered a policy that is substantially similar to the high-risk plan at a premium in excess of that insurance, or
- Have been previously enrolled in another state's high-risk insurance pool.

Premium cap: The cap for the first year of the policy may not exceed 150 percent of the standard rate. For future years, this figure may increase to 175 percent of the standard rate.

Waiting Period for Preexisting Conditions and Waiver of Waiting Period

- *Waiting period for preexisting conditions:* Coverage is excluded during a six-month period following the effective date of coverage for any condition for which diagnosis, care, or treatment was recommended or received during the six months immediately preceding enrollment medical advice.
- *Waiver of waiting period:* MCHIRP will limit its exclusion in treating a preexisting condition to three months if the insured was covered under another policy that was terminated for a reason other than his or her fault. A preexisting condition waiting period also does not apply to an insured who is federally eligible.

Coverage

The Mississippi Risk Pool Plan is a major medical plan that offers deductibles of $1,000 medical/$250 pharmacy, $2,000 medical/$500 pharmacy, or $3,000 medical/$500 pharmacy. Benefits are generally covered on an 80/20 co-pay basis, and there is no limit on out-of-pocket amount under the plan. Benefits include

- Outpatient/doctor visits
- Inpatient care/hospital services
- Prescription drug coverage: Nonpreferred brands at 50 percent of allowable charge; brand names at 80 percent of allowable charge; and generic drugs at 100 percent of allowable charge
- Physical therapy: $5,000 per calendar year with a lifetime maximum of $20,000
- Durable medical equipment

Lifetime benefit: $500,000 ($100,000 annual)

■ MISSOURI

Organization Administering Insurance and Contact:

Organization: Missouri Health Insurance Pool
State contact:
Missouri Health Insurance Pool
1831 Chestnut Street
St. Louis, MO 63103
800-645-8346
816-395-2583

Eligibility Criteria and Premium Cap

An individual may be eligible for coverage through the MHIP if he or she is a Missouri resident who meets any of the following requirements:

- Was turned down for individual health insurance or HMO coverage within the past six months because of medical condition or health history
- Was offered individual health insurance or HMO coverage within the past six months at a premium that exceeded 300 percent of the standard rate for individual coverage
- Was previously covered under another state's medical high-risk pool and applies for MHIP coverage within 30 days of becoming a Missouri resident
- Was previously covered under an employer's group health plan under COBRA but attained the maximum coverage period
- Was involuntarily terminated from prior health coverage for any reason (for example, an insurance carrier chose to withdraw from the Missouri market)

Premium cap: The cap may not be less than 150 percent or more than 200 percent of the standard rate.

Waiting Period for Preexisting Conditions and Waiver of Waiting Period

- *Waiting period for preexisting conditions:* Coverage is excluded during the first 12 months following the effective date of coverage for any condition for which medical care, diagnosis, or advice was recommended or received or should have been sought by an ordinarily prudent person during the six-month period immediately preceding the effective date of coverage.
- *Waiver of waiting period:* There is a waiver of the waiting period if it has already been satisfied under any prior coverage that was involuntarily terminated, and if

coverage is applied for within 60 days or if conversion rates are 300 percent of the standard rate set by the pool.

Coverage

MHIP offers individual coverage through four major medical plans, which differ only in the amount of the annual deductible and out-of-pocket maximums. The plans offered are structured as PPOs with a co-insurance of 20 percent for in-network provider services and 50 percent for out-of-network provider services. The following summarizes the deductible amounts offered with corresponding out-of-pocket maximums:

	Plan I	Plan II	Plan III	Plan IV
In-network deductible	$500 per year	$1,000 per year	$2,500 per year	$5,000 per year
Out-of-network deductible	$1,000 per year	$2,000 per year	$5,000 per year	$10,000 per year
Out-of-pocket maximum*	$2,500 per year + deductible	$5,000 per year + deductible	$5,000 per year + deductible	$5,000 per year + deductible

* The maximum applies only to services received by in-network providers.

Benefits include:

■ Outpatient care/doctor visits
■ Inpatient care/hospital, including surgery
■ Prescription drug coverage
■ Skilled nursing care
■ Home health visits
■ Physical therapy

Lifetime benefit: $1,000,000

■ MONTANA

Organization Administering Insurance and Contact:

Organization: Montana Comprehensive Health Association
State contact:
    Montana Comprehensive Health Association
    c/o Blue Cross/Blue Shield of Montana
    560 North Park Avenue
    Helena, MT 59604
    406-444-8537
    800-447-7828

Note: Effective May 1, 2004: Due to funding availability limitations, enrollment is temporarily closed. The MCHA will continue to accept applications for this program, but qualifying applicants will be placed on a waiting list, with future enrollment being on a first-come, first-served basis. Qualified applicants may choose to enroll in the MCHA plan for which they qualify while waiting to be enrolled in the Premium Assistance Program. The MCHA Board anticipates that the program will be reopened in the future.

Eligibility Criteria and Premium Cap

An individual is eligible if he or she meets the following criteria:

- Is a resident of the state;
- Has received one of the following by at least two insurers within six months prior to application:
    - Rejection for disability or health insurance; or
    - A restrictive rider or preexisting condition limitation;
- Has a specified major illness; and
- Is not eligible for any other health insurance coverage.

An individual also qualifies by meeting the standards of federal eligibility.

Premium cap: The Board of the Montana Comprehensive Health Association has set the premium cap at 200 percent of the average of top five insurers of individual plans.

Waiting Period for Preexisting Conditions and Waiver of Waiting Period

- *Waiting period for preexisting conditions:* Benefits are not covered for any preexisting condition for 12 months following the effective date of coverage. A preexisting condition is defined as any condition for which medical advice, care, or treatment was recommended or received from a medical practitioner during the five-year period preceding the effective date of coverage.
- *Waiver of waiting period:* The waiting period does not apply to newborn children or children placed for adoption. Otherwise, creditable coverage will apply if
    - Applicant did not voluntarily cancel coverage;
    - Application was made within 30 days of the most recent coverage; and
    - All other options for insurance (including COBRA) have been exhausted.
- There is no waiting period for applicants who meet the standards set for federal eligibility.

Coverage

If the applicant is federally eligible, he or she will have the choice of two portability plans and the Traditional Plan. Otherwise, only the Traditional Plan is available.

The Traditional Plan is structured as a PPO with a co-payment of 20 percent and a deductible of $1,000, with a maximum out-of-pocket, including the deductible, of $5,000. Benefits include:

- Hospital services
- Physician services
- Physical therapy
- Ambulance services
- Durable medical equipment
- Home health care

■ NEBRASKA

Organization Administering Insurance and Contact

Organization: Nebraska Comprehensive Health Insurance Pool (CHIP)

State contact:

>CHIP Customer Service Center
Blue Cross/Blue Shield of Nebraska
P.O. Box 3248
Main Post Office
Omaha, NE 68180-0001
402-390-1814
877-348-4304

Eligibility Criteria and Premium Cap

To be eligible to purchase CHIP, you must either

- Be a resident of the state for at least six-months; and
- Have been rejected for health insurance coverage within the last six months from an insurer licensed in Nebraska for medical reasons; or
- Have been offered, within six months prior to application, health insurance subject to a restrictive rider limiting coverage for a preexisting medical condition; or

■ Have been offered coverage at a rate exceeding the premium rate for pool coverage; or

■ Have a diagnosis of one of several specified medical conditions that automatically qualifies the applicant for coverage; or

■ Be a Nebraska resident for any length of time; and

■ Have been covered for 18 months by prior creditable coverage under a group employer, governmental, or church plan; and

■ Not be eligible for Medicare or Medicaid; and

■ Not had most recent coverage terminated because of nonpayment of premiums or fraud; and

■ If offered COBRA coverage and exhausted it, the premium for the continuation coverage is higher than the CHIP premium.

Premium cap: The Nebraska Comprehensive Health Insurance Pool has set the premium cap at 135 percent of the rate for comparable coverage.

Waiting Period for Preexisting Conditions and Waiver of Waiting Period

■ *Waiting period for preexisting conditions:* Charges and expenses listed as a benefit in the policy will not be allowed if incurred during the first six months following the effective date of coverage for any condition that has manifested itself or for which medical advice, care, or treatment was recommended or received during the six-month period preceding coverage.

■ *Waiver of waiting period:* A waiver of the waiting period is possible if one of the following has occurred:

  – Health coverage was involuntarily terminated because of the withdrawal by the insurer from the state, the bankruptcy or insolvency of the employer or employer trust fund, or the employer ceasing to provide any group health plan for all of its employees. The applicant must be eligible for CHIP coverage and must apply for the preexisting waiver within 60 days after the termination of prior coverage. The applicant cannot be eligible for a conversion policy or a continuation of coverage policy under federal or state law.

  – Medicaid coverage ended within six months of the effective date of CHIP coverage.

  – The applicant received medical assistance through the Medically Handicapped Children's Program within six months of the effective date of CHIP coverage.

- The applicant was an organ transplant recipient terminated from Medicare within six months of the effective date of CHIP coverage.

- The applicant had a health continuation policy under state or federal law (COBRA) that was terminated or involuntarily terminated for any reason other than nonpayment of premium. Application for CHIP coverage must be made within 90 days of the end of prior coverage.

- The applicant qualifies for CHIP because of maintaining 18 months of prior creditable coverage under a group, governmental, or church plan and applies for CHIP coverage within 63 days of termination of the most recent creditable coverage.

Coverage

The Comprehensive Health Insurance Pool offers two types of plans: a PPO and a major medical plan. The PPO plan has a selection of deductibles from $250 to $5,000 with co-insurance of 20 percent for in-network charges and 30 percent for out-of-network charges. The major medical plan has deductibles from $500 to $10,000 with a co-insurance of 20 percent. Coverage offered in both plans includes

- Hospital room and board
- Physician services
- Physical, occupational, and speech therapy
- X-ray and laboratory exams
- Medical supplies
- Prescription drugs
- Home health care
- Skilled nursing care

Lifetime benefit: $1,000,000

■ NEW HAMPSHIRE

Organization Administering Insurance and Contact

Organization: New Hampshire Health Plan
State contact:
    CBA/EPBA
    37 Industrial Drive, Suite E
    Exeter, NH 03833
    877-888-NHHP (6447)

Eligibility Criteria and Premium Cap

Participants must be residents of New Hampshire to apply for NHHP coverage. Eligibility depends on their meeting any of the following requirements:

- Have applied for individual health insurance and been declined due to health or medical condition
- Have applied for individual health insurance and been offered coverage similar to that available from NHHP but at a higher premium
- Have a medical condition that is on the list of prequalifying conditions (see below)
- Be federally eligible and not eligible for, have not been offered, or have exhausted continuation coverage under COBRA or a similar program
- Be a resident dependent of an individual covered by NHHP (or a resident family member of a child covered by NHHP)
- Have been offered health insurance with a rider excluding coverage for a specified condition

If you are a New Hampshire resident and produce evidence of a specified prequalified medical condition, you do not have to apply to another insurance company before applying for NHHP coverage.

Premium cap: The premium cap is 125–150 percent of comparable coverage

Waiting Period for Preexisting Conditions and Waiver of Waiting Period

- *Waiting period for preexisting conditions:* During the first nine months NHHP polices will not pay benefits for certain preexisting conditions.
- *Waiver of waiting period:* NHHP will credit time under prior creditable coverage if that coverage was continuous (with no break over 62 days) to a date not more than 63 days prior to receipt of the application. To get credit toward satisfaction of the preexisting condition period, applicants must submit a certificate or other evidence of prior creditable coverage.

Coverage

NHHP offers two indemnity plans, with deductibles of $2,000 or $3,000, and three managed care plans, with deductibles ranging from $1,000 to $5,000 (higher for out-of-network). They also offer an option that qualifies as a "high-deductible health plan" under federal Health Savings Account (HSA) provisions. Co-insurance is 20 percent for indemnity plans, 20 percent for in-network MCO services, and 40 percent for out-of network MCO services. Services covered include

- Hospital confinement
- Diagnostic services
- Skilled nursing
- Rehabilitation
- Physician visits (routine physical exams not covered in indemnity plans)
- Home health care
- Medical equipment and supplies

Lifetime benefit: $2,000,000

■ NEW MEXICO

Organization Administering Insurance and Contact

Organization: New Mexico Medical Insurance Pool (NMMIP)
State contact:
New Mexico Blue Cross/Blue Shield
P.O. Box 27630
Albuquerque, NM 87125-7630
800-432-0750, option 4
505-816-5671

Eligibility Criteria and Premium Cap

Participant must be a resident of New Mexico and

- Have received notice of rejection of coverage for substantially similar health insurance; or
- Have received notice that the rate applied to his or her coverage will exceed the premiums imposed on the comprehensive insurance as to its $500 deductible plan; or
- Have received a notice of reduction or limitation of coverage, including a restrictive rider that excludes benefits for a condition for longer than 12 months that is specific to the applicant; or

■ Have lost coverage from an individual plan due to the insurer having stopped offering such coverage or because it no longer sells health insurance in New Mexico.

A resident is also eligible if he or she meets the criteria for federal eligibility.

Premium cap: The premium is capped at 125 percent of the standard rate for comparable coverage.

Waiting Period for Preexisting Conditions and Waiver of Waiting Period

■ *Waiting period for preexisting conditions:* The coverage under the comprehensive insurance plan excludes charges or expenses incurred during the first six months following the effective date of coverage if the condition manifested itself or if medical advice, care, or treatment was recommended or received within six months preceding the effective date of coverage.

■ *Waiver of waiting period:* The waiting period is waived if similar exclusions have been satisfied under any prior health insurance coverage that was involuntarily terminated and the application for comprehensive coverage is made within 31 days following the involuntary termination. In that case, such coverage will be effective from the date that the prior coverage was terminated. Individuals who are federally eligible are not subject to a waiting period.

Coverage

NMMIP provides six regular plans, each with a different deductible and out-of-pocket maximum, and one Medicare carve-out. Deductibles range from $500 to $10,000 a year, depending on the plan selected. Out-of-pocket expenses range from $2,500 to $5,000. After the deductible is paid, the percentage covered by the insurer ranges from 80 to 100 percent. Benefits include

■ Hospital room and board
■ Basic medical and surgical services
■ Professional services provided by a physician for the treatment or diagnosis of an illness or injury
■ Rental or purchase of durable medical equipment
■ Private-duty nursing service (limited to $10,000 of covered expenses per person per calendar year)
■ Prescription drugs (subject to a 25 percent per prescription co-payment)

- Skilled nursing facility services up to 100 days per person per calendar year
- Home health visits: 100 medically necessary visits per year from a licensed home health agency
- Physical therapy

Lifetime benefit: No maximum lifetime benefit

▪ NORTH DAKOTA

Organization Administering Insurance and Contact

Organization: Comprehensive Health Association of North Dakota (CHAND)
State contact:
Administrative Board
Blue Cross/Blue Shield of North Dakota
4510 13th Avenue SW
Fargo, ND 58121-0001
800-737-0016
701-277-2271

Eligibility Criteria and Premium Cap

A participant must

- Have been a resident of the state of North Dakota continuously for six months;
- Be under the age of 65; and
- Within the last six months have
  - Written evidence of rejection by one insurer; or
  - Been offered coverage by an insurer that is subject to a rider substantially restricting benefits for specific conditions.

A resident is also eligible if he or she meets the criteria for federal eligibility.

Premium cap: The premium may not exceed 135 percent of the standard rate for comparable coverage.

Waiting Period for Preexisting Conditions and Waiver of Waiting Period

- *Waiting period for preexisting conditions:* Coverage will not be provided for services, supplies, or charges received during the first 180 days of the policy (270 days for maternity benefits) for the treatment of any preexisting condition that was diagnosed or treated within 90 days prior to the effective date of the policy.

■ *Waiver of waiting period:* A waiting period of 180 consecutive days will be reduced by the number of days the qualifying previous plan was in effect. A reduction in this waiting period is allowed only if there is no break in coverage greater than 62 days between the two plans. Applicants who are federally eligible are not subject to a waiting period.

Coverage

The plan offered is structured as a medical plan with a co-payment of 20 percent after the deductible is met. The deductibles offered are $500 and $1,000. The co-insurance maximum for the calendar year for the plan offering a $500 deductible is $2,500; the plan subject to a $1,000 deductible has a co-insurance maximum of $2,000. Once the out-of-pocket amount exceeds $3,000 for either plan (deductible plus co-insurance), the benefit amount for covered services for the remainder of the calendar year is 100 percent. The services offered under the CHAND plan include

■ Hospitalization and in-hospital medical care
■ Surgical services
■ Physical therapy
■ Outpatient care/doctor visits
■ Prescription drug coverage
■ Skilled nursing services
■ Home health visits
■ Rental or purchase of durable medical equipment

Lifetime benefit: $1,000,000

■ OKLAHOMA

Organization Administering Insurance and Contact

Organization: Oklahoma Health Insurance High Risk Pool (OHRP)
State contact:
    EPOCH Group
    6717 Shawnee Mission Parkway
    Overland, KS 66202
    405-741-8434
    800-255-6065

Eligibility Criteria and Premium Cap

An individual applying for coverage under the Medical Eligibility Program must meet the following criteria:

▪ Be a legal resident of Oklahoma for a period of at least 12 months;

▪ Have been rejected by two insurers for coverage substantially similar to the high-risk insurance offered in the state because of a health condition;

▪ Have been accepted for health insurance that excludes coverage for the insured's preexisting condition;

▪ Have been quoted an individual policy rate substantially higher than the OHRP rate; or

▪ Have a specified prequalified medical condition

A resident is also eligible if he or she meets the criteria for federal eligibility.

Premium cap: The cap has been set at 150 percent of the average standard rate for comparable coverage.

Waiting Period for Preexisting Conditions and Waiver of Waiting Period

▪ *Waiting period for preexisting conditions:* A high-risk policy may contain provisions excluding coverage during a period of 12 months following the effective date of the policy as to a participant's preexisting condition, as long as

– The condition manifested itself within a period of six months before the effective date of coverage; or

– Medical advice or treatment for the condition was recommended or received within a period of six months before the effective date of coverage.

▪ *Waiver of waiting period:* The 12-month waiting period will be waived if the participant was covered under another policy that provided hospital, medical, or surgical benefits, and coverage under that policy terminated less than 63 days prior to coverage beginning under the OHRP policy. Individuals who are federally eligible are not subject to a waiting period.

Coverage

The plan offered is structured as a PPO with a co-payment of 20 percent of allowable charges for in-network provider services and 40 percent of allowable charges for out-of-network provider services. Six deductibles are offered, ranging from $500 to $7,500. Coverage includes

- Hospital services
- Professional services for the diagnosis and treatment of injuries, illnesses, or conditions other than dental
- Prescription drugs
- Services of a home health agency
- Nursing facility services
- Physical therapy

Lifetime benefit: $500,000

■ OREGON

Organization Administering Insurance and Contact

Organization: Oregon Medical Insurance Pool (OMIP)
State contact:
    Regence Blue Cross/Blue Shield of Oregon
    P.O. Box 1271
    Portland, OR 97207
    503-225-6620
    800-848-7280

Eligibility Criteria and Premium Cap

One must be an Oregon resident and meet any of the following medical or portability requirements:

Medical requirements: Within the last six months:
- Have been declined individual health insurance coverage due to health reasons;
- Have one or more of the specified medical conditions;
- Have been offered individual health insurance coverage that contained a restrictive waiver that substantially reduced the coverage offered by excluding coverage for a specific medical condition;
- Have been offered individual health insurance coverage but was limited by the choice of plans the carrier was willing to offer due to a specific medical condition.

Portability requirements: To be eligible under the portability criteria, one must apply within 63 days of losing COBRA, losing portability coverage from another insurer in Oregon, or losing group health benefits coverage because of moving from another state to Oregon. Coverage must be continuous from the termination of prior coverage. The following conditions must also be met:

- COBRA benefits have been exhausted.
- No COBRA or portability coverage was available through previous plan.
- Applicant eligible for Oregon portability coverage but moved from the prior insurance carrier's service area.
- Applicant has portability coverage, but insurance carrier no longer serves the area of residency.
- Applicant moved to Oregon and have been continuously covered by health insurance for 18 or more months, with no single gap in coverage greater than 63 days and the last coverage was group coverage.

A resident is also eligible if he or she meets federal eligibility.

Premium cap: The premium is initially set at 125 percent of the standard rate for comparable coverage.

Waiting Period for Preexisting Conditions and Waiver of Waiting Period

▪ *Waiting period for preexisting conditions:* Preexisting conditions will not be covered for the first six months of enrollment unless credit is granted toward the waiting period.

▪ *Waiver of waiting period:* A participant may receive credit toward the waiting period if he or she had prior health coverage, was involuntarily terminated, and an application for OMIP was made within 60 days of termination. Individuals who are federally eligible are not subject to a waiting period.

Coverage

Oregon has four different plans to choose from, all of which are preferred provider plans. Therefore, there is a benefit to using providers within the plan network. These four plans offer a range of deductibles: $500, $750, $1,000, and $1,500. Maximum out-of-pocket costs range from $1,000 to $6,000 in-network, and $2,000 to 12,000 out-of-network. Benefits provided under the plans include

▪ Hospitalization
▪ Doctor visits
▪ Skilled nursing care

- Prescription drugs (no out-of-pocket maximum)
- Rental or purchase of durable medical equipment
- Emergency room
- Physical therapy
- Surgery

Lifetime benefit: $1,000,000

■ SOUTH CAROLINA

Organization Administering Insurance and Contact

Organization: South Carolina Health Insurance Pool
State contact:
    Blue Cross/Blue Shield of South Carolina
    P.O. Box 61173
    Columbia, SC 29260-1173
    800-868-2500, ext. 42757

Eligibility Criteria and Premium Cap

The participant must be a resident of South Carolina for 30 days and have experienced any of the following:

- Refusal of health insurance by any insurer for health reasons
- Refusal of insurance except with a reduction of coverage for a preexisting condition exceeding 12 months
- Refusal of comparable insurance coverage except at a rate exceeding 150 percent of the pool rate

An individual may also qualify for coverage if he or she meets the standards of federal eligibility.

Premium cap: The premium charged may not exceed 200 percent of the standard rate for comparable coverage.

Waiting Period for Preexisting Conditions and Waiver of Waiting Period

- *Waiting period for preexisting conditions:* Coverage under the plan excludes charges incurred during the first six months following the effective date of coverage as to any condition (a) which, during the six-month period immediately preceding the effective date of coverage, manifested itself in a manner that would cause an ordinarily prudent person to seek diagnosis, care, or treatment; or (b) for which medical care, advice, or treatment was recommended or received.

▪ *Waiver of waiting period:* The waiting period is waived if satisfied under the previous insurance for which coverage was involuntarily terminated or if the applicant is federally eligible.

Coverage

Health insurance pool benefits are comparable to those of many private insurance plans. The pool pays 80 percent of allowed charges for covered hospital inpatient and outpatient treatment, physician services, prescription drugs, and certain other medical care. Persons covered by the pool pay the remaining 20 percent and must meet a $500 deductible each year before the pool coverage begins to pay. Monthly premiums are determined by the person's age and sex. There is no family coverage under the pool. Each policy is for individual coverage. The benefits provided in the plans include:

▪ Inpatient hospital expense
▪ Outpatient care/doctor visits (after deductible is met)
▪ Surgery
▪ Home health visits
▪ Prescription drug coverage
▪ Physical therapy
▪ Durable medical equipment

Lifetime benefit: $1,000,000

▪ SOUTH DAKOTA

Organization Administering Insurance and Contact

Organization: South Dakota Risk Pool
State contact:
    Attn: South Dakota Risk Pool
    c/o Bureau of Personnel
    500 East Capitol Avenue
    Pierre, SD 57501
    605-773-3148

Eligibility Criteria and Premium Cap

The be eligible for the South Dakota Risk Pool, an applicant must

- Be a resident of South Dakota
- Apply within 63 days of losing prior coverage;
- Have at least 12 months of continuous creditable coverage
- Have used up COBRA or state continuation coverage
- Have not had one's most recent coverage terminated due to nonpayment of premiums or fraud
- Not be covered under a group health plan, Medicare, Medicaid, or any other form of health insurance

Premium cap: The cap is set by the state at 150 percent of the standard rate for comparable coverage.

Waiting period for Preexisting Conditions and Waiver of Waiting Period

Since South Dakota accepts only people into the program who have recent creditable coverage, there is no waiting period for coverage of preexisting conditions

Coverage

South Dakota offers four plans for their high-risk pool. Deductibles for these plans range from $1,000 to $10,000. One plan, at the $3,000 level, qualifies as a health savings account (HSA) option. Out-of-pocket costs for these plans, excluding pharmacy, have limits ranging from $3,250 to $12,250. Following payment of the deductible, the plan pays 75 percent of medical service and pharmaceutical costs. Benefits include

- Hospitalization
- Medical services
- Physical, occupational, and speech therapy
- Prescription drugs
- Home health services
- Skilled nursing facility

Lifetime benefit: $1,000,000

■ TEXAS

Organization Administering Insurance and Contact

Organization: Texas Health Insurance Risk Pool
State contact:
    Texas Health Insurance Risk Pool
    P.O. Box 6089
    Abilene, TX 79608
    888-398-3927

Eligibility Criteria and Premium Cap

An individual is eligible for high-risk insurance if he or she is under the age of 65, is a legal resident of Texas for at least 30 days, has been a United States citizen or a permanent resident of the United States for at least three continuous years, and provides evidence of one of the following:

■ Notice of rejection or refusal by an insurance company to issue substantially similar health coverage due to health reasons;

■ An offer by an insurer or HMO to issue individual health coverage providing substantially similar coverage at a premium rate greater than the current Health Pool rate;

■ Certification from a salaried representative of an insurance company or agent that the applicant is unable to obtain substantially similar individual coverage because of the applicant's medical condition; or

■ An offer by either an HMO or an insurer to issue a policy that excludes a medical condition or conditions.

An individual may also qualify for coverage if he or she meets standards of federal eligibility.

Premium cap: The first-year premium is capped between 125 and 150 percent of the standard rate for comparable individual health insurance and 200 percent of the standard rate for renewal years.

Waiting Period for Preexisting Conditions and Waiver of Waiting Period

■ *Waiting period for preexisting conditions:* Coverage is excluded during a 12-month period following the effective date of coverage for any condition for which medical advice, care, or treatment was recommended or received during the six months immediately preceding enrollment.

■ *Waiver of waiting period:* The preexisting condition limitation does not apply if an individual was continuously covered for a period of 12 months under other health coverage that was in effect up to a date not more than 63 days before the participant's effective date of coverage through the Health Pool. Credit is given for the time the insured was covered under any prior health insurance that was in effect at any time during the 12-month period before the effective date of Health Pool coverage. Individuals who are federally eligible are not subject to a waiting period.

Coverage

Texas offers three plans in their high-risk pool with deductibles ranging from $1,000 to $5,000. Co-insurance for network services is 20 and 40 percent for non-network services. The co-insurance maximum for preferred providers is $3,000. There is no maximum for non-preferred providers. The benefits provided in the plan include

■ Hospital

■ Doctor visits

■ Prescription drugs

■ Home health care

■ Skilled nursing facility

■ Physical, occupational, and speech therapy

■ Durable medical equipment

Lifetime benefit: $1,500,000

■ UTAH

Organization Administering Insurance and Contact

Organization: Utah Comprehensive Health Insurance Pool (UCHIP)

State contact:

UCHIP
P.O. Box 30270
Salt Lake City, UT 84130
801-333-5573

Eligibility Criteria and Premium Cap

An individual is eligible for the insurance offered by UCHIP if he or she meets the following criteria:

■ Has resided in Utah for at least 12 months

■ Pays the established premium

■ Applied for comprehensive health coverage not more than 30 days after being denied coverage by a private individual insurer

■ In the event of termination of a similar type of insurance from another state because the applicant is now a resident of Utah, has applied for the UCHIP policy within 31 days from the date of cancellation

An individual may also qualify for coverage if he or she meets standards of federal eligibility.

Waiting Period for Preexisting Condition and Waiver of Waiting Period

■ *Waiting period for preexisting conditions:* Coverage is excluded during a six-month period following the effective date of the insurance for any condition for which diagnostic care or treatment was recommended or received during the six-month period immediately preceding enrollment.

■ *Waiver of waiting period:* A waiver is effective if the individual applies for an HIP plan within 31 days of losing his or her prior coverage. If the previous insurance was from another state high-risk pool, the application period is extended to 63 days. Individuals who are federally eligible are not subject to a waiting period.

Coverage

HIPUtah has three plans. Covered benefits are the same under all three plans, but the annual deductible varies. Deductibles range from $500 to $2,500. After a deductible, HIP pays 80 percent of covered services by participating providers and 60 percent of covered services provided by nonparticipating providers. The maximum out-of-pocket liability per plan year is $1,000 in co-insurance plus the annual deductible. After this maximum is reached, HIPUtah will pay 100 percent of covered services by participating providers and 95 percent of covered services provided by nonparticipating providers. Benefits include

■ Inpatient hospital services

■ Outpatient care/doctor services

- Physical therapy
- Prescription drugs
- Durable medical equipment
- Home health services
- Medical supplies
- Laboratory, radiological, and other diagnostic tests

Lifetime benefit: $1,000,000; $250,000 annually

▪ WASHINGTON

Organization Administering Insurance and Contact

Organization: Washington State Health Insurance Pool (WSHIP)
State contact:
    Benefit Management Incorporated
    P.O. Box 1090
    Great Bend, KS 67530
    800-877-5187

Eligibility Criteria and Premium Cap

The applicant must

- Be a resident of the state of Washington; and
- Have proof of rejection for health insurance for medical reasons; or
- Reside in a county in Washington in which individual health benefit plans are not marketed to the general public by a member insurance carrier.
- In the case of a Medicare-eligible applicant, have one of the following:
  - Health insurance with a restrictive rider;
  - Health insurance with a preexisting condition limitation; or
  - Health insurance with an up-rated premium.

An individual may also qualify for coverage if he or she meets the standards of federal eligibility.

Premium cap: The premium may not exceed 150 percent of the standard rate for comparable insurance except in the case of a managed care policy, when the premium cannot exceed 125 percent of the standard rate.

Waiting Period for Preexisting Conditions and Waiver of Waiting Period

■ *Waiting period for preexisting conditions:* Coverage is excluded during a period of six months following the effective date of coverage for a condition for which medical advice, care, or treatment was recommended or received during the six months preceding enrollment.

■ *Waiver of waiting period:* The waiting period for preexisting conditions will be waived if similar exclusions have been satisfied under any prior health insurance, provided that such coverage had been terminated no more than 63 days from the date the individual applies for WSHIP. Individuals who are federally eligible are not subject to a waiting period.

Coverage

WSHIP offers three comprehensive plans, each with a pharmacy benefit. One plan is a standard indemnity plan with a deductible of $500, $1,000, or $3,000. Out-of-pocket costs will be lower if services are received from a provider who is part of the First Choice network. The second plan is a preferred provider plan with a choice of a $500, $1,000, $2,500, or $5,000 deductible. Out-of-pocket costs range from $1,000 to $10,000 for in-network care and $2,000 to $15,000 for out-of-network services. The third plan is for persons enrolled in Parts A and B of Medicare who have health insurance with a restrictive rider, preexisting condition exclusion, or up-rated premium. The benefits in the plans include

■ Semi-private hospital room and board and any other hospital services and supplies
■ Professional services including surgery and treatment of injuries
■ Prescription drugs
■ Home health services and skilled nursing care
■ Physical therapy
■ Durable medical equipment
■ Diagnostic X-ray and ambulance

Lifetime benefit: $1,000,000

■ WEST VIRGINIA

Organization Administering Insurance and Contact

Organization: Access WV
State contact:
    Access WV
    P.O. Box 50540
    Charleston, WV 25305
    866-445-8491

Eligibility Criteria and Premium Cap

Eligible individuals are those who have been a resident of West Virginia for at least 30 days and

- Are not eligible to receive coverage under a group insurance plan offered either by employer or their spouse's;
- Are not eligible for medical coverage under a federal or state program including Medicare, Medicaid, and WVCHIP; and
- Are not residents of a public institution (i.e., a federal or state correctional institution or a Veteran's Home).

Applicants must also have experienced at least one of the following:

- Been rejected for health insurance coverage by a carrier selling health insurance in West Virginia within the last six months; or
- Received coverage from a carrier selling health insurance in West Virginia that offers less coverage or similar coverage at a greater price than AccessWV; or
- Be eligible under HIPAA; or
- Have a preexisting, severe, or chronic medical condition.

Waiting Period for Preexisting Conditions and Waiver of Waiting Period

- *Waiting period for preexisting conditions:* Some enrollees will be subject to a six-month preexisting condition waiting period before claims for services related to their health condition will be paid by the plan.
- *Waiver of waiting period:* Persons who have federal eligibility under HIPAA will not have a preexisting condition exclusionary period.

Coverage

Applicants are able to purchase either single or family coverage. There are three different plans, A, B, and C. Deductibles and out-of-pocket maximums vary depending on the plan chosen. For example, the single in-network deductible is $400 in Plan A but $2,000 in Plan C. The single in-network out-of-pocket maximum ranges from $2,000 in Plan A to $3,000 in Plan C. Benefits covered include

- Hospital
- Physician services
- Outpatient services
- Home care
- Prescription drugs
- Rehabilitation

Lifetime benefit: $1,000,000; $200,000 annually

■ WISCONSIN

Organization Administering Insurance and Contact

Organization: Wisconsin Health Insurance Risk Sharing Plan (HIRSP)
State contact:
HIRSP
1751 West Broadway
P.O. Box 8961
Madison, WI 53708
800-828-4777

Eligibility Criteria and Premium Cap

Participants must

- Be a resident of Wisconsin for a period of at least 30 days
- Not be eligible for employer-sponsored group insurance
- Not be eligible for Wisconsin Medicaid

■ If not federally eligible and under 65, have received one of the following within the past nine months:

  – Notice of rejection or cancellation from one or more health insurers;

  – Notice of a reduction or limitation in health insurance coverage that substantially reduces coverage compared to coverage available to persons considered standard risks;

  – Notice of an increase in a health insurance premium that exceeds the premium then in effect for the insured person by 50 percent or more, unless the increase applies to substantially all of the insurer's health policies then in effect; or

  – Notice of premium rate increase for health insurance applied for but not yet in effect. (This notice must be from one or more insurers and again be exceeded by at least 50 percent.)

An individual is also eligible if he or she meets the criteria for federal eligibility.

Premium cap: The premium is capped at 200 percent of the standard rate for comparable health insurance.

Waiting Period for Preexisting Conditions and Waiver of Waiting Period

■ *Waiting period for preexisting conditions:* Conditions diagnosed or treated in the six months preceding the policy date will not be covered for the first six months that a participant is covered by the plan.

■ *Waiver of waiting period:* The waiting period for preexisting conditions will be waived if similar exclusions have been satisfied under any prior health insurance, provided that such coverage had been terminated no more than 63 days from the date that the individual applies for HIRSP. Individuals who are federally eligible are not subject to a waiting period.

Coverage

Wisconsin offers the following two plans:

■ Plan 1: This plan is for individuals who are not Medicare eligible and provides the insured a choice of either a $1,000 or $2,500 deductible with an annual out-of-pocket maximum of $2,000 or $3,500, respectively. The options have identical coverage and differ only in the amounts of premiums, deductibles, and co-insurance.

▪ Plan 2: This plan is for individuals who are Medicare eligible. The insurance is subject to an annual $500 deductible, and the insured is not required to pay any co-insurance.

Both plans offer the following coverage:

▪ Hospital services
▪ Basic medical/surgical services
▪ Prescription drugs
▪ Skilled nursing care
▪ Home health visits
▪ Physical therapy
▪ Diagnostic/X-ray

Lifetime benefit: $1,000,000

▪ WYOMING

Organization Administering Insurance and Contact

Organization: Wyoming Health Insurance Pool

State contact:

Wyoming Health Insurance Pool
4000 House Avenue
P.O. Box 2419
Cheyenne, WY 82003
307-634-1393
800-442-2376

Eligibility Criteria and Premium Cap

The participant must be a resident of the state and have proof of

▪ Rejection or refusal to issue health insurance for health reasons by one insurer;
▪ Refusal of health insurance except at a rate exceeding the pool rate; or
▪ Refusal of health insurance except with a reduction or exclusion of coverage for a preexisting condition for which reduction or exclusion is more restrictive than that provided by the pool.

An individual may also qualify for coverage if he or she meets the standards of federal eligibility.

Premium cap: The premium is not to exceed 200 percent of the standard market rate.

Waiting Period for Preexisting Conditions and Waiver of Waiting Period

■ *Waiting period for preexisting condition:* Coverage is excluded during a 12-month period following the effective date of coverage for a condition for which medical advice, care, diagnosis, or treatment was recommended or received during the six months immediately preceding enrollment.

■ *Waiver of waiting period:* The preexisting condition limitation does not apply if the individual was continuously covered for a period of 12 months under other health insurance that was in effect up to a date that was not more than 90 days before the participant's effective date of coverage through the state health insurance pool. An individual who is federally eligible is not subject to a waiting period.

Coverage

Two options are available from the Wyoming Health Insurance Pool: the Brown Plan and the Gold Plan. Coverage under both plans includes Type A, Type B, and Type C benefits and is differentiated by certain benefits and how they are paid. Type A benefits include high-cost expenses such as inpatient hospitalization, outpatient and office surgery, and ambulance services. Type B benefits include the smaller, less costly items and services such as outpatient prescriptions, outpatient medical care, office calls, and physical therapy. Type C benefits include maternity care, including prenatal care, delivery, and postnatal care.

Out-of-pocket costs include deductibles and co-insurance. Once the out-of-pocket maximum has been met, the plan will pay 100 percent of reasonable and customary charges for covered services. Benefits covered include

■ *Physician services* (including inpatient and outpatient surgery). Neither plan imposes a deductible, and 80 percent of reasonable and customary charges are paid until the out-of-pocket maximum is met. Thereafter, 100 percent of reasonable and customary expenses are covered.

■ *Ambulance.* Neither plan imposes a deductible; 80 percent of reasonable and customary charges are paid until the out-of-pocket maximum is met. Thereafter, 100 percent of reasonable and customary expenses are covered, subject to contract maximums.

- *Other covered services* (including prescription drug coverage, durable medical equipment, physical therapy, and physician office calls). The Brown Plan is subject to a $2,000 annual deductible per individual. Once the deductible has been met, the insurer pays 70 percent of reasonable and customary expenses until the out-of-pocket maximum is reached. Thereafter, 100 percent of reasonable and customary charges are covered. The Gold Plan is subject to a $1,000 annual deductible per individual. Once the deductible has been met, the insurer pays 70 percent of reasonable and customary expenses until the out-of-pocket maximum has been reached. Thereafter, 100 percent of reasonable and customary charges are covered.

- *Out-of-pocket maximum.* The out-of-pocket maximum is $4,000 for the Brown Plan and $2,000 for the Gold Plan.

Lifetime benefit: $600,000 in the Gold Plan; $350,000 in the Brown Plan.

APPENDIX 1

INSURANCE DIRECTORY: STATE TELEPHONE NUMBERS (2007)

■ ALABAMA

- **Department of Insurance**, 201 Monroe Street, Suite 1700, Montgomery, AL 36104; 334-269-3550
- **Alabama Health Insurance Plan** (high-risk insurance), State Employees Insurance Board, 201 Monroe Street, P.O. Box 304900, Montgomery, AL 36130-4900; 877-619-2447
- **Medicaid**, 501 Dexter Avenue, Montgomery, AL 36103; 334-242-5000
- **State Health Insurance Assistance Program (SHIAP)**: Educates and assists Medicare beneficiaries, those eligible for Medicare, and caregivers about Medicare, Medicaid, Medigap, pharmacy assistance programs, and other issues related to health insurance benefits. 770 Washington Avenue, Suite 470, Montgomery, AL 36130; 800-243-5463 or 334-242-5743

■ ALASKA

- **Division of Insurance**, Consumer Services Office, 550 West 7th Street, 15th Floor, Anchorage, AK 99501; 800-467-8725 or 907-269-7900
- **Medicaid, Division of Medical Assistance**, P.O. Box 110660, Juneau, AK 99811-0660; 800-780-9972 or 907-465-3355

■ **Alaska Comprehensive Health Insurance** (ACHI) (high-risk insurance), 2015 16th Street, Great Bend, KS 67530; 888-290-0616

■ **Alaska Medicare Information, Division of Senior Services:** Educates and assists Medicare beneficiaries, those eligible for Medicare, and caregivers about Medicare, Medicaid, Medigap, pharmacy assistance programs, and other issues related to health insurance benefits. 3601 C Street, Suite 310, Anchorage, AK 99503-5209; 800-478-6065 (in-state) or 907-269-3680

■ ARIZONA

■ **Department of Insurance,** Consumer Service Division, 2910 North 44th Street, Suite 210, Phoenix, AZ 85018; 602-912-8400

■ **Medicaid,** 801 East Jefferson Street, Phoenix, AZ 85034-2246; 800-526-3022

■ **State Health Insurance Assistance Program (SCHIAP):** Educates and assists Medicare beneficiaries, those eligible for Medicare, and caregivers about Medicare, Medicaid, Medigap, pharmacy assistance programs, and other issues related to health insurance benefits. 1789 West Jefferson Street, Phoenix, AZ 85007; 800-432-4040 or 602-542-6595

■ ARKANSAS

■ **Department of Insurance,** Consumer Services Division, 1200 West Third Street, Little Rock, AR 72201; 501-371-2600

■ **Medicaid, Arkansas Department of Human Services,** Donoghey Plaza, Seventh and Main Street, P.O. Box 1347, Little Rock, AR 72203; 501-682-8292

■ **Comprehensive Health Insurance Plan** (high-risk insurance), Arkansas Comprehensive Health Insurance Pool, P.O. Box 419, Little Rock, AR 72203; 501-370-2659 or 800-285-6477

■ **State Health Insurance Information Program (SHIIP):** Educates and assists Medicare beneficiaries, those eligible for Medicare, and caregivers about Medicare, Medicaid, Medigap, pharmacy assistance programs, and other issues related to health insurance benefits. Arkansas Insurance Department, 1200 West Third Street, Little Rock, AR 72201-1904; 800-224-6330 or 501-371-2782

■ CALIFORNIA

■ **Department of Managed Care, California HMO Help Center:** Serves residents enrolled in HMOs and Blue Shield PPOs (serves mostly privately insured consumers); helps resolve problems with medical care, prescription drugs, preventive testing, and mental health services; assists with questions regarding the complaint process and health care rights; and provides education. 980 Ninth Street, Suite 500, Sacramento, CA 95814; 888-HMO-2219

■ **State of California Department of Insurance**, 300 Capital Mall, Suite 1700, Sacramento, CA 95814; 916-492-3500 or 800-927-4357

■ **Medi-Cal**, P.O. Box 997413, Sacramento, CA 95899; 916-636-1980

■ **Managed Risk Medical Insurance Program** (high-risk insurance), Managed Risk Insurance Board, P.O. Box 2769, Sacramento, CA 95812-2769; 800-289-6574

■ **Health Insurance Counseling and Advocacy Program (HICAP)**: Educates and assists Medicare beneficiaries, those eligible for Medicare, and caregivers about Medicare, Medicaid, Medigap, pharmacy assistance programs, and other issues related to health insurance benefits. 1300 National Drive, Suite 200, Sacramento, CA 95834; 1-800-434-0222 or 914-491-7500

■ COLORADO

■ **Department of Regulatory Agencies, Colorado Division of Insurance**, 1560 Broadway, Suite 850, Denver, CO 80202; 800-930-3745 or 303-894-7499

■ **Medicaid, Colorado Department of Health Care Policy and Financing**, 1570 Grant Street, Denver, CO 80203; 303-866-2993 or 800-221-3943

■ **CoverColorado** (high-risk insurance), 425 South Cherry Street, Suite 160, Glendale, CO 80246; 877-461-3811

■ **State Health Insurance Information Program (SHIIP)**: Educates and assists Medicare beneficiaries, those eligible for Medicare, and caregivers about Medicare, Medicaid, Medigap, pharmacy assistance programs, and other issues related to health insurance benefits. Colorado Division of Insurance, 1560 Broadway, Suite 850, Denver, CO 80202; 1-800-554-9181 (in-state)

■ CONNECTICUT

■ **Department of Insurance**, P.O. Box 816, Hartford, CT 06142; 860-297-3800

■ **Medicaid, Division of Social Services**, 25 Sigourney Street, Hartford, CT 06106; 860-424-4908 or 800-842-1508

■ **Connecticut Health Reinsurance Association** (high-risk insurance), 100 Great Meadow Road, Suite 704, Weathersfield, CT 06109; 800-842-0004

■ **CHOICES, Connecticut Department of Social Services:** Educates and assists Medicare beneficiaries, those eligible for Medicare, and caregivers about Medicare, Medicaid, Medigap, pharmacy assistance programs, and other issues related to health insurance benefits. Division of Elderly Services, 25 Sigourney Street, Hartford, CT 06106; 800-994-9422 (in-state) or 860-424-5274

■ **Office of Healthcare Advocate:** Serves residents enrolled in managed care, providers, and employers. P.O. Box 1543, Hartford, CT 06144; 1-866-HMO-4446

■ DELAWARE

■ **Department of Insurance,** 841 Silver Lake Boulevard, Rodney Building, Dover, DE 19904; 800-282-8611 or 302-739-4251

■ **Medicaid, Division of Social Services,** 1901 North Dupont Highway, New Castle, DE 19720; 800-372-2022 or 302-255-9500

■ **ELDERInfo,** Delaware Insurance Department: Educates and assists Medicare beneficiaries, those eligible for Medicare, and caregivers about Medicare, Medicaid, Medigap, pharmacy assistance programs, and other issues related to health insurance benefits. 841 Silver Lake Boulevard, Dover, DE 19904; 800-336-9500

■ DISTRICT OF COLUMBIA

■ **Insurance Administration,** 810 First Street N.E., Suite 701, Washington, DC 20002; 202-727-8000

■ **Medicaid, Department of Medical Assistance,** 824 North Capital Street N.E., Washington, DC 20002; 202-742-5506 or 888-557-1116

■ **Health Insurance Counseling Project (HICP):** Educates and assists Medicare beneficiaries, those eligible for Medicare, and caregivers about Medicare, Medicaid, Medigap, pharmacy assistance programs, and other issues related to health insurance benefits. GWU National Law Center, Building A–BV, 2136 Pennsylvania Avenue, Washington, DC 20052; 202-739-0668

■ FLORIDA

■ **Department of Insurance,** 200 East Gaines Street, Tallahassee, FL 32399-0300; 800-342-2762 or 850-413-2806

■ **Bureau of Medicaid**, P.O. Box 13000, Tallahassee, FL 32317; 850-488-3560 (The telephone number is to the State's Directors Office for the Bureau of Medicaid. Personnel from this office will provide telephone numbers and addresses to county offices.)

■ **Florida Comprehensive Health Association** (high-risk insurance), 1210 East Park Avenue, Tallahassee, FL 32301; 850-309-1200 (Note that the office is not processing new applications. Only those individuals currently insured under the program may have their coverage renewed.)

■ **Servicing Health Insurance Needs for Elders (SHINE)**: Educates and assists Medicare beneficiaries, those eligible for Medicare, and caregivers about Medicare, Medicaid, Medigap, pharmacy assistance programs, and other issues related to health insurance benefits. Department of Elder Affairs, 4040 Esplanada Way, Tallahassee, FL 32399-7000; 800-963-5337 or 850-414-2060

■ **Statewide Provider and Subscriber Assistance Program**: Serves residents enrolled in managed care and helps resolve grievance between managed care entities and their subscribers. 2727 Mahan Drive, Suite 339, Ft. Knox, FL 32308; 1-888-419-3459

■ GEORGIA

■ **Department of Insurance**, 2 Martin Luther King Jr. Drive, Atlanta, GA 30344; 800-656-2704 or 404-656-2070

■ **Medicaid**, 2 Peachtree NW, Floor 39, Atlanta, GA 30303; 866-322-4260 or 770-570-3300

■ **Health Insurance Counseling Assistance and Referral for the Elderly (HICARE)**: Educates and assists Medicare beneficiaries, those eligible for Medicare, and caregivers about Medicare, Medicaid, Medigap, pharmacy assistance programs, and other issues related to health insurance benefits. 2 Peachtree NW, Suite 9-210, Atlanta, GA 30303; 800-669-8387 or 404-657-5437

■ HAWAII

■ **Commerce and Consumer Affairs**, Department of Insurance Division, 335 Merchant Street, Honolulu, HI 96813; 808-586-2790

■ **Medicaid**; Department of Human Services, c/o Ms. Aileen Hiramatsu, Administrator, P.O. Box 339, Honolulu, HI 96809; 808-587-3521

■ **Executive Office on Aging:** Educates and assists Medicare beneficiaries, those eligible for Medicare, and caregivers about Medicare, Medicaid, Medigap, pharmacy assistance programs, and other issues related to health insurance benefits. 250 South Hotel Street, Suite 406, Honolulu, HI 96813-2831; 1-888-875-9229

■ IDAHO

■ **Department of Insurance,** Consumer Assistance Office, 700 West State Street, Third Floor, Boise, ID 83720; 208-334-4250

■ **Medicaid,** Idaho Department of Health and Welfare, 3232 Elder Street, Boise, ID 83705; 208-334-5747 or 1-877-200-5441

■ **High Risk Reinsurance Pools Plan,** Idaho Department of Insurance, 700 West State Street, Third Floor, Boise, ID 83720-0043; 208-334-4250 or 800-721-3272

■ **State Health Insurance Assistance Program aka Senior Health Insurance Benefits Advisers (SHIBA):** Educates and assists Medicare beneficiaries, those eligible for Medicare, and caregivers about Medicare, Medicaid, Medigap, pharmacy assistance programs, and other issues related to health insurance benefits. 700 West State Street, Third Floor, Boise, ID 83720-0043; 800-247-4422

■ ILLINOIS

■ **Department of Insurance,** Springfield office: 320 West Washington Street, Springfield, IL 62767; 217-785-5516. Chicago office: 100 West Randolph Street, Suite 15-100, Chicago, IL 60601; 312-814-5559 or 877-527-9431

■ **Medicaid, Department of Public Aid,** 201 South Grand Avenue, Springfield, IL 62763; 217-782-1200 or 866-468-7543

■ **Illinois Comprehensive Health Insurance** (high-risk insurance), 320 West Washington, Suite 300, Springfield, IL 62701; 866-851-2751

■ **Office of Consumer Health Insurance:** Established on January 1, 2000, the office will answer questions concerning health insurance, explain provisions contained in a specific health plan, explain the legal rights guaranteed to a health care consumer, and assist with complaints against an insurer. 320 West Washington Street, Springfield, IL 62767; 877-527-9431 (in-state) or 217-782-4515

■ **Senior Health Insurance Program (SHIP):** Educates and assists Medicare beneficiaries, those eligible for Medicare, and caregivers about Medicare,

Medicaid, Medigap, pharmacy assistance programs, and other issues related to health insurance benefits. 320 West Washington Street, Springfield, IL 62767-0001; 800-548-9043 or 217-785-9021

▪ INDIANA

- **Department of Insurance**, 311 West Washington Street, Suite 300, Indianapolis, IN 46204; 800-622-4461 or 317-232-2385
- **Indiana Family and Social Service Administration**: Information on State of Indiana Medicaid, 402 West Washington Street, Indianapolis, IN 46207; 800-889-9949 or 317-233-4455
- **Indiana Comprehensive Health Insurance Association** (high-risk insurance), P.O. Box 33730, Indianapolis, IN 46203; 800-552-7921, 317-614-2000, or 317-614-2133
- **Senior Health Insurance Information Program (SHIIP)**: A source for information about Medicare, Medicare supplement insurance, Medicare Advantage, long-term care insurance, prescription coverage, and low-income assistance. 311 West Washington Street, Suite 300, Indianapolis, IN 46204; 800-452-4800

▪ IOWA

- **Division of Insurance**, Health Insurance, 330 Maple Street, Des Moines, IA 50319; 877-955-1212 or 515-281-5523
- **Medicaid, Division of Medical Services**, Hoover State Office Building, Fifth Floor, Des Moines, IA 50319; 800-338-8366 or 515-327-5121
- **Division of Insurance, Iowa Consumer Affairs Bureau**: This bureau handles consumer complaints and questions from the public. The unit conducts investigations and, when necessary, brings actions against insurance companies. 330 Maple Street, Des Moines, IA 50319; 515-281-4241
- **Health Insurance Plan of Iowa (HIPIOWA)** (high-risk insurance), P.O. Box 1090, Great Bend, KS 67530; 877-793-6880
- **Senior Health Insurance Information Program (SHIIP)**: Resource for information on Medicare, Medicare supplement insurance, long-term care insurance, and other health insurance issues. 330 Maple Street, Des Moines, IA 50319; 800-351-4664

■ KANSAS

■ **Department of Insurance, Consumer Insurance Affairs Bureau**, 420 Southwest Ninth Street, Topeka, KS 66612; 800-432-2484 or 785-296-3071

■ **Medicaid**, 915 Southwest Harrison Street, D.S.O.B., Room 652, Topeka, KS 66612; 785-274-4200 or 800-766-9012

■ **Kansas Health Insurance Association** (high-risk insurance), P.O. Box 1090, Great Bend, KS 67530; 800-362-9290

■ **Senior Health Insurance Counseling for Kansas (SHICK)**: A source for information on Medicare, Medicare supplement insurance, long-term care insurance, and other insurance subjects that concern older Kansans, Wichita, KS 67202; 800-860-5260

■ KENTUCKY

■ **Department of Insurance**, 215 West Main Street, P.O. Box 517, Frankfort, KY 40602; 502-564-6027 or 800-595-6053

■ **Medicaid, Department of Health Services**, P.O. Box 2110, Frankfort, KY 40602; 502-564-4321 or 800-635-2570

■ **Division of Consumer Protection and Education**: A division assisting consumers in complaints against insurance companies. P.O. Box 517, Frankfort, KY 40602; 800-595-6053 (in-state) or 502-564-6034

■ **Kentucky Access** (high-risk insurance), P.O. Box 33707, Indianapolis, IN 46203-0707; 866-405-6145

■ **Benefits Counseling Section of the Office of Aging**: Helps residents understand Medicare and/or Medicaid coverage and supplemental insurance, understand and compare supplemental policies and plans, fill out prescription drug discount program applications, and apply for public benefits. 275 East Main Street, Frankfort, KY 40621; 877-293-7447

■ LOUISIANA

■ **Department of Insurance**, P.O. Box 94214, Baton Rouge, LA 70804; 800-259-5300 or 225-342-5423

■ **Medicaid, Department of Health and Hospital Services**, P.O. Box 91278, Baton Rouge, LA 70821; 225-342-5774 or 888-342-6207

■ **Louisiana Health Insurance Association** (high-risk insurance), P.O. Drawer 83880, Baton Rouge, LA 70884-3880; 800-736-0947

■ **Senior Health Insurance Information Program (SHIIP)**: A source for answers to health insurance questions on topics including supplemental and long-term care insurance policy comparison, assistance with claims, Medicare-contracted HMOs, Medicare supplement (Medigap) Insurance, and the Medicare appeals process. P.O. Box 94214, Baton Rouge, LA 70804; 800-259-5301

■ MAINE

■ **Bureau of Insurance**, State Office Building, Station 34, Augusta, ME 04333; 800-300-5000 or 207-624-8401

■ **Medicaid, Bureau of Medical Services**, 11 State House Station, Augusta, ME 04333; 800-977-6740, option 2, or 207-624-7539

■ **Maine Health Insurance Counseling Program**: Provides information and answers questions about Medicare, Medicare-approved drug discount cards, MaineCare, Medigap, and other programs and benefits that supplement Medicare. 11 State House Station, 442 Civic Center Drive, Augusta, ME, 04333 877-353-3771

■ MARYLAND

■ **Insurance Administration, Life and Health Division**, 525 St. Paul Place, Baltimore, MD 21202; 800-492-6116 or 410-468-2090

■ **Medicaid, Recipient Relations Unit**, 201 West Preston Street, Room L-9, Baltimore, MD 21201; 800-492-5231 (in-state) or 410-767-5800

■ **Maryland Health Insurance Plan** (high-risk insurance), 509 Progress Drive, Linthicum, MD, 21090; 866-780-7105

■ **Senior Health Insurance Assistance Program**: A source of information on Medicare, Medigap, assistance for disabled Medicare beneficiaries (under age 65), Medicare Advantage plans, long-term care insurance, and medical assistance programs. 301 West Preston Street, Suite 1007, Baltimore, MD 21204; 800-243-3425 or 410-767-1100

■ MASSACHUSETTS

■ **Division of Insurance**; Consumer Health Line, 1 South Station, Boston, MA 02110; 617-521-7794

▪ **Medicaid, Customer Service, Division of Medical Assistance**, 600 Washington Street, Boston, MA 02111; 800-325-5231

▪ **MassHealth**: A comprehensive health insurance and premium assistance program for senior citizens and disabled individuals. 300 Ocean Avenue, Revere, MA 02151; 800-841-2900

▪ **Senior Health Insurance Needs for Elders (SHINE)**: A source for answers to health insurance questions on topics including Medicare Part A and Part B, Medigap insurance, Medicare HMOs, retiree insurance plans, prescription drug programs, Medicaid, Medicare assistance programs (QMB, SLMB, and QI), and other programs for people with limited resources. 1 Ashburton Place, Boston, MA 02108; 800-243-4636, option 2

▪ MICHIGAN

▪ **Department of Commerce, Division of Insurance**, P.O. Box 30220, Lansing, MI 48909; 517-373-0220 or 877-999-6442

▪ **Medicaid**, Family Independence Agency, P.O. Box 30037, Lansing, MI 48909; 517-373-3740 or 800-642-3195

▪ **Michigan Medicare Medicaid Assistance Program**: A source for information regarding supplemental (Medigap) insurance evaluation and comparison, billing concerns, managed care (Medicare Advantage) options, long-term care insurance evaluation and comparison, Medicaid assistance (including application), Medicare appeals process, and prescription drug assistance (including EPIC). 6105 West St. Joseph Highway, Suite 209, Lansing, MI 48917-4850; 800-803-7174

▪ MINNESOTA

▪ **Department of Commerce, Insurance Enforcement Division**: The Insurance Enforcement Division regulates health insurance except in matters involving HMOs.) 85 East Seventh Place, St. Paul, MN 55101; 651-296-5769

▪ **Department of Health**: Regulates matters pertaining to HMOs. 121 East Seventh Place, Metro Square Building, Suite 400, St. Paul, MN 55101-2117; 800-657-3916 (in-state) or 651-282-5608

▪ **Medicaid, Department of Human Services**, 444 Lafayette Road, St. Paul, MN 55101; 800-333-2433 or 651-297-3933

▪ **Minnesota Comprehensive Health Association** (high-risk insurance), 5775 Wayzata Boulevard., St. Louis Park, MN 55416; 952-593-9609

■ **Minnesota SHIP/ Senior Link Age Line:** A source for information on health insurance, including Medicare, long-term care insurance, prescription drug coverage, and financial planning. 444 Lafayette Road, St. Paul, MN 55164 ; 800-333-2433

■ MISSISSIPPI

■ **Insurance Department, Consumer Services Division:** The telephone numbers are for general insurance information and filing a complaint against an insurance company. 501 North West Street, Suite 1001 Woolfolk State Office Building, Jackson, MS 39201; 800-562-2957 or 601-359-3569

■ **Medicaid Division,** 239 North Lamar Street, Jackson, MS 39201; 800-421-2408 or 601-359-6050

■ **Mississippi Comprehensive Health Insurance Risk Pool Association** (high-risk insurance), Risk Pool Association, P.O. Box 13748, Jackson, MS 39236; 601-899-9967 or 888-820-9400

■ **Mississippi Insurance and Counseling Program (MICAP)** A source of information to help residents understand Medicare benefits, organize doctor and hospital bills, file Medicare appeals, review Medicare supplemental Insurance, evaluate Medicare+Choice or HMO options, understand Medicaid eligibility, and explore long-term care options. 750 North State Street, Jackson, MS 39202; 800-948-3090

■ MISSOURI

■ **Department of Insurance; Consumer Affairs Division,** 301 West High Street, Jefferson City, MO 65102; 800-726-7390 or 573-751-4126

■ **Medicaid; Division of Medical Services,** 221 West High Street, Jefferson City, MO 65102; 573-751-4815 or 800-392-2161

■ **Missouri Health Insurance Pool** (high-risk insurance), 1831 Chestnut Street, St.Louis, MO 63103; 800-645-8346 or 816-395-2583

■ **Missouri CLAIM Program (Community Leaders Assisting the Insured of Missouri):** A source for answers to health insurance questions regarding Medicare eligibility, enrollment and claims forms, employment and retirement health benefits, supplemental insurance policies, Medicare Advantage options, such as HMOs and PPOs, Medicare-approved discount cards and Medicare Part D, long-term care planning, and public benefit programs. 3425 East Constitution Court, Jefferson City, MO 65109; 800-390-3330

■ MONTANA

■ **State Auditor's Office, Insurance Division** (issues relating to health insurance), 840 Helena Avenue, Helena, MT 59601; 800-332-6148 or 406-444-2040

■ **Medicaid,** 1400 Broadway, Helena, MT 59604; 800-362-8312 or 406-444-4540

■ **Montana Comprehensive Health Association** (high-risk insurance), c/o Blue Cross/Blue Shield of Montana, 560 North Park Avenue, Helena, MT 59604; 406-444-8537 or 800-447-7828 (Enrollment was temporarily closed in 2006 but applications continue to be accepted.)

■ **Montana Senior and LTC Division (SHIP):** A statewide source of program information for beneficiaries of Medicare, Medicaid, Medicare supplemental policies, long-term care insurance, and other heath insurance benefits. 111 North Sanders Street, Helena, MT 59604; 800-551-3191

■ NEBRASKA

■ **Department of Insurance, Life and Health Division,** 941 O Street, Suite 400, Lincoln, NE 68508; 877-564-7323 or 402-471-2201

■ **Medicaid, Department of Health and Human Services,** P.O. Box 95044, Lincoln, NE 68509; 800-430-3244 or 402-471-3121

■ **Nebraska Comprehensive Health Insurance Pool** (high-risk insurance), Blue Cross/Blue Shield of Nebraska, P.O. Box 3248, Main Post Office, Omaha, NE 68180-0001; 402-390-1814 or 877-348-4304

■ **Nebraska State Health Insurance Information, Counseling and Assistance Program (NICA):** A source for answers to health insurance questions on topics such as Medicare and Medicaid benefits, eligibility and claims, as well as Medicare supplement, long-term carem and group health insurance. 941 O Street, Lincoln, NE 68508; 800-234-7119

■ NEVADA

■ **Department of Business and Industry, Division of Insurance,** 788 Fairview Drive, Suite 300, Carson City, NV 89701; 775-687-4270 or 800-992-0900

■ **Medicaid, Nevada Department of Human Resources,** 1100 East William Street, Carson City, NV 89701; 775-684-7200

■ **State Health Insurance Assistance Program (SHIP),** Division of Aging Services: A source for answers to health insurance questions on topics including eligibility for Medicare entitlements, benefits, limitations, Medicaid (qualified Medicare beneficiary (QMB) and specified low-income Medicare beneficiary (SLMB), fee-for-service plans, and coordinated care plans (HMOs). West Sahara Street, Las Vegas, NV 89102; 800-307-4444

■ NEW HAMPSHIRE

■ **Department of Insurance, Consumer Division**, 21 South Fruit Street, Suite 14, Concord, NH 03301; 800-852-3416 or 603-271-2261

■ **Medicaid Client Services, Consumer Assistance Office**, 129 Pleasant Street, Concord, NH 03301; 800-852-3345, ext. 8166 or 603-271-4322

■ **New Hampshire Health Plan** (high-risk pool), CBA/EPBA, 37 Industrial Drive, Suite E, Exeter, NH 03833; 877-888-6447

■ **Health Insurance Counseling Education and Assistance Services (HICEAS)**: A source of information regarding Medicare, Medicare supplement insurance, Medicare managed care, Medicare+Choice, QMB/SLMB, and long-term care insurance. P.O. Box 2338, Concord, NH 03302-2338; 800-852-3388 (in-state) or 603-225-9000

■ NEW JERSEY

■ **Department of Banking and Insurance, Life and Health Section**, 20 West State Street, Trenton, NJ 08625; 609-777-4443 or 800-446-7467

■ **Medicaid, Division of Medical Assistance and Health Services**, P.O. Box 712, Trenton NJ 08625-0712; 609-588-2600 or 800-356-1561

■ **Department of Banking and Insurance, Consumer Protection**, P.O. Box 329, Trenton, NJ 08640-0329; 609-292-5316

■ **Department of Health and Senior Services, State Health Insurance Assistance Program (SHIP)**: A source of information on health insurance coverage and benefits that affect Medicare beneficiaries; P.O. Box 360, Trenton, NJ 08625; 800-792-8820

■ NEW MEXICO

■ **New Mexico Department of Insurance, Life and Health Division**, PERA Building, Room 519, 1120 Paseo de Peralta, Santa Fe, NM 87501; 800-947-4722 or 505-827-4601

■ **Medicaid, Human Services Department Medical Assistance Division Help Desk**, P.O. Box 2348, Santa Fe, NM 87504-2348; 888-997-2583 (in-state) or 505-827-3100

■ **New Mexico Medical Insurance Pool**, P.O. Box 27630, Albuquerque, NM 87125-7630; 800-432-0750 or 505-816-5671

■ **New Mexico Benefits Counseling Program/Aging and LTC Services Department**: A source of information regarding Medicare/Medicaid/Medigap benefits, claim denial appeals, HMO information and locations, nursing home and home health care coverage, SSI, and other public benefits programs. 2550 Cerrillos Road, Santa Fe, NM 87505; 800-432-2080

■ NEW YORK

■ **Department of Insurance**: The following are regional addresses and telephone numbers that may be used for consumer complaints against insurance companies and inquiries on health insurance. 25 Beaver Street, New York, NY 10004; 212-480-2289 or 800-342-3736

■ **Medicaid Help line**, 99 Washington Avenue, Albany, NY 12210; 518-486-9057 or 800-541-2831

■ **New York Health Insurance Information Counseling & Assistance Program**: A source to help people understand and make choices regarding Medicare, Medicaid, Medicare managed care, private insurance (including Medigap and long-term care insurance), and related public benefits. 2 Empire State Plaza, Agency Building #2, Albany, NY 12223; 800-701-0501

■ NORTH CAROLINA

■ **Department of Insurance**, P.O. Box 26387, 430 North Salisbury Street, Raleigh, NC 27603; 800-662-7777 or 919-733-3058

■ **Medicaid Assistance, Department of Health and Human Services**, 2501 Mail Service Center, Raleigh, NC 27698; 919-855-4100

■ **Senior Health Insurance Information Program (SHIIP)**: A source for answers to health insurance questions regarding Medicare, Medicare supplement insurance and long-term care insurance. 111 Seaboard Avenue, Raleigh, NC 27604; 800-443-9354

■ NORTH DAKOTA

■ **Department of Insurance, Health Insurance Hotline**, 600 East Boulevard, 5th Floor, Bismarck, ND 58505; 800-247-0560 or 701-328-2440

- Medicaid Assistance, Department of Human Services Medical Services Division, 600 East Boulevard, Department 325, Bismarck, ND 58505; 800-755-2604 or 701-328-2321

- Comprehensive Health Association of North Dakota (CHAND) (high-risk insurance), Blue Cross/Blue Shield of North Dakota, 4310 13th Avenue S.W., Fargo, ND 58121; 800-737-0016 or 701-277-2271

- Senior Health Insurance Counseling (SHIC): Helps individuals understand Medicare bills and statements, compare and understand Medicare supplement and long-term care insurance, compare and understand Medicare Part D, evaluate insurance coverage, and assist with claims or appeals. 600 East Boulevard, Bismarck, ND 58505; 888-575-6611

■ OHIO

- Department of Insurance, Managed Care Division, 2100 Stella Court, Columbus, OH 43215; 614-644-2658 or 800-686-1526

- Medicaid Division, Department of Human Services, 30 East Broad Street, Columbus, OH 43266; 614-728-3288 or 800-324-8680

- Department of Insurance, Consumer Hotline, 2100 Stella Court, Columbus, OH 43215; 800-686-1526 (office to file complaints)

- Ohio Senior Insurance Information Program (OSHIIP): A source for answers to health insurance questions on topics including Medicare, Medicaid, Medicare Advantage plans, Medicare supplement insurance, and other health insurance-related topics. 2100 Stella Court, Columbus, OH 43215; 800-686-1578

■ OKLAHOMA

- Department of Insurance, Life and Health Division, 2401 Northwest 23rd Street, Suite 28, Oklahoma City, OK 73107; 800-522-0071 or 405-521-2828

- Medicaid, Department of Social Services, 4545 North Lincoln Boulevard,Oklahoma City, OK 73105; 405-522-7171 or 800-522-0310

- Oklahoma Health Insurance High Risk Pool, EPOCH Group, 6717 Shawnee Mission Parkway, Overland, KS 66202; 405-741-8434 or 800-255-6065

- Senior Health Insurance Counseling Program (SHICP): A source for answers to health insurance questions on topics including Medicare, Medicaid, Medicare supplements, Medicare Advantage, long-term care, and other related health coverage plans for Medicare beneficiaries. 2401 Northwest 23rd Street, Suite 28, Oklahoma City, OK 73107; 800-763-2828

■ OREGON

■ **Department of Consumer and Business Services, Life and Health Insurance Division**, 350 Winters Street N.E., Room 440, Salem, OR 97301; 888-877-4894 or 503-947-7980

■ **Oregon Health Plan, Adult and Family Service Division (Medicaid)**, 500 Summer Street N.E., Salem, OR 97310; 800-527-5772 or 503-945-5772

■ **Oregon Medical Insurance Pool** (high-risk insurance), P.O. Box 1271, Portland, OR 97207; 800-848-7280 or 503-225-6620

■ **Senior Health Insurance Benefits Assistance Program (SHIBA):** Educates, assists, and serves as advocates for people with Medicare. Helps people with Medicare understand their rights and options in health insurance, so that they can make informed choices. 250 Church Street S.E., Salem, OR 97301; 800-722-4134

■ PENNSYLVANIA

■ **Department of Insurance**, Consumer Information and Complaint, 1326 Strawberry Square, Harrisburg, PA 17120; 717-783-0442 or 877-881-6388

■ **Department of Public Welfare, Medicaid Recipient Hotline**, 1401 North Seventh Street, Harrisburg, PA 17105; 800-692-7462 or 717-787-1870

■ **Apprise Health Care and Counseling, Department of Aging:** Answers questions about Medicare, Medicare supplement insurance, Medicaid, and long-term care insurance. 555 Walnut Street, Harrisburg, PA 17101; 800-783-7067

■ RHODE ISLAND

■ **Department of Business Regulations Insurance Division Office of Life and Health**, 233 Richmond Street, Suite 233 Providence, RI 02903; 401-222-5466

■ **Department of Human Services, Medicaid**, 600 New London Avenue, Cranston, RI 02921; 401-462-5300 or 800-984-8989

■ **Rhode Island Senior Health Insurance Program:** A resource for older adults and adults with disabilities to help them understand their health care options. Benjamin Rush Building #55, 35 Howard Avenue, Cranston, RI 02920; 401-462-3000

■ SOUTH CAROLINA

■ **Department of Insurance, Life, Accident, and Health Division**, 300 Arbor Lake Drive, Suite 1200, Columbia, SC 29223; 800-768-3467 or 803-737-6212

■ **Department of Social Services, Medical (Medicaid) Division**, P.O. Box 8206, Columbia, SC 29202; 803-898-2500 or 888-549-0820

■ **South Carolina Health Insurance Pool** (high-risk insurance), Blue Cross/Blue Shield of South Carolina, P.O. Box 61173, Columbia, SC 29260-1173; 800-868-2500, ext. 42757

■ **South Carolina Bureau of Senior Services**: A source for answers to health insurance questions on topics including Medicaid, Medigap, and long-term care insurance coverage. Jefferson Square Building, Columbia, SC 29202; 800-868-9095

■ SOUTH DAKOTA

■ **Division of Insurance**, 445 East Capital Avenue, Pierre, SD 57501; 605-773-4104

■ **Department of Social Services, Medicaid**, 700 Governors Drive, Pierre, SD 57501; 605-773-3495 or 800-452-7691

■ **South Dakota Risk Pool** (high-risk insurance), 500 East Capital Avenue, Pierre, SD, 57501 605-773-3148

■ **Adult Services and Aging**: Educates Medicare beneficiaries and their families on Medicare and Medicare Advantage issues, as well as private health insurance policies like long-term care insurance and Medicare supplemental insurance. 700 Governors Drive, Pierre, SD 57501; 800-536-8197

■ TENNESSEE

■ **Department of Insurance, Consumer Insurance Services Office**, 500 James Robertson Parkway, 4th Floor, Nashville, TN 37243; 800-342-4029 (in-state) or 615-741-6007

■ **Department of Human Services (Medicaid)**, 310 Great Circle Road, Nashville, TN 37243; 866-311-4287

■ **Tennessee Commission of Aging and Disability**: Provides free and objective counseling and assistance to persons with questions or problems regarding Medicare and other related health insurances. 500 Deaderick Street, Nashville, TN 37243; 877-801-0044

■ TEXAS

■ **Department of Insurance, Consumer Protection Division**, 333 Guadalupe Street, Austin, TX 78701; 800-578-4677 or 512-463-6464

▪ **Department of Human Services, Medicaid**, 4900 North Lamar Boulevard, Austin, TX 78701; 888-834-7406 or 512-424-6500

▪ **Texas Health Insurance Risk Pool** (high-risk insurance) P.O. Box 6089, Abilene, Texas 79608; 888-398-3927

▪ **Texas Department of Aging and Disability Services**: Assists people who receive Medicare benefits by providing benefits counseling to those 60 plus years of age and Medicare beneficiaries, including those with disabilities, regardless of age. 701 West 51st Street, Austin, TX 78751; 800-252-9240

▪ UTAH

▪ **Insurance Department, Consumer Service Assistance**, 3110 State Office Building, Salt Lake City, UT 84114; 800-439-3805 or 801-538-3800

▪ **Insurance Department, Health Insurance Complaint Division**, 310 State Office Building, Salt Lake City, UT 85114; 801-538-3805 (Salt Lake City only) or 800-350-6242 (for remaining areas of the state)

▪ **Department of Health, Medicaid**, 288 North 1460 West, Salt Lake City, UT 84114; 801-538-6155 or 800-662-9651

▪ **Utah Comprehensive Health Insurance Pool**, P.O. Box 30270, Salt Lake City, UT 84130; 801-333-5573

▪ **State Health Insurance Assistance Program (SHIP)**, aka Aging and Adult Services): A source for information regarding Medicare A and B, Medicare supplemental coverage, and long-term care insurance. 120 North 200 West Street, Salt Lake City, UT 84103; 800-541-7735

▪ VERMONT

▪ **Department of Banking, Insurance, Securities, and Health Care Administration**, 89 Main Street, Drawer 20, Montpelier, VT 05620; 802-828-3301

▪ **Vermont Division of Health Care Administration**: Information provided on health plans, health insurance, and health care services available in Vermont. 89 Main Street, Third Floor, Montpelier, VT 05620; 800-631-7788 (in-state) or 802-828-2900

▪ **Department of Health and Human Services, Medicaid**, 103 South Main Street, Waterbury, VT 05676; 800-250-8427 or 802-879-5900

■ **Office of Health Care Ombudsman**: Separate state office providing information on patient rights and consumer complaints against health insurers) 264 North Winooski Avenue, Burlington, VT 05402; 800-917-7787 (in-state) or 802-863-2316

■ **Vermont Area Agency on Aging of Vermont**: A resource to help with questions or problems with Medicare or other health insurance, including the Vermont state programs. 1166 Portland Street, St. Johnsbury, VT 05819; 800-642-5119

■ VIRGINIA

■ **State Corporation Commission, Bureau of Insurance**, 1300 East Main Street, Richmond, VA 23219; 800-552-7945 or 804-371-9694

■ **Department of Social Services, Medical Assistance Services** (Medicaid), 600 East Broad Street, Richmond VA 23 219; 804-786-7933

■ **Virginia Insurance Counseling and Assistance Program**: A source for assistance with insurance filing and billing, as well as sorting through complicated statements and notices. 1610 Forest Avenue, Richmond, VA 23229; 800-552-3402

■ WASHINGTON

■ **State Insurance Commission, Office of Consumer Protection and Information**, P.O. Box 40255, Olympia, WA 98504; 800-562-6900 or 360-725-7000

■ **Department of Health and Social Services, Medical Assistance Customer Service Center (Medicaid)**, 1011 Plum Street, Olympia, WA 98504; 800-562-3022

■ **Washington State Health Insurance Pool** (high-risk insurance), Benefit Management Incorporated, P.O. Box 1090, Great Bend, KS 67530; 800-877-5187

■ **State Health Insurance Benefits Advisor Program (SHIBA)**: Helps people of all ages with questions about health insurance, health care access, and prescription access. P.O. Box 45600, Olympia, WA 98504; 800-562-6900

■ WEST VIRGINIA

■ **Commission of Insurance, Health Insurance Consumer Division**, 1124 Smith Street, Room 309, Charleston, WV 25301; 304-558-3354 or 888-879-9842

▪ **Department of Health and Human Resources, Medicaid**, 350 Capitol Street, Charleston, WV 25301; 304-558-1700

▪ **Access West Virginia** (high-risk pool), P.O. Box 50540, Charleston, WV 25305, 866-445-8491

▪ **State Health Insurance Network (SHINE)**, aka Bureau of Senior Services): Provides counseling, assistance, and advocacy relating to Medicare, Medicare Advantage, Medicare assistance (buy-in) programs, private health insurance (including Medicare supplement [Medigap] and long-term care policies), and related health coverage plans. Capitol Building, 1900 Kanawha Boulevard, Charleston, WV 25305; 877-987-4463

▪ WISCONSIN

▪ **Insurance Commission**, 125 South Webster Street, GEFIII, Madison, WI 53702; 608-267-1233 or 800-236-8517

▪ **Medicaid**, 1 West Wilson Street, Madison, WI 53701; 800-362-3002 or 608-221-5720

▪ **Wisconsin Health Insurance Risk Sharing Plan (HIRSP)** (high-risk insurance), Wisconsin Health Insurance Risk Sharing Plan, 1751 West Broadway, Madison, WI 53708; 800-828-4777

▪ **Wisconsin State Health Insurance Assistance Program**: A source of information regarding Medicare, Medicare supplement insurance, SSI, Social Security, medical assistance, and consumer problems. 1402 Pankratz Street, Madison, WI 53704 800-242-1060

▪ WYOMING

▪ **Department of Insurance** (consumer information or complaints), 122 West 25th Street, Herschler Building, Third Floor East, Cheyenne, WY 82002; 800-438-5768 or 307-777-7401

▪ **Department of Health**, Medicaid Division, 147 Hathaway Boulevard, Cheyenne, WY 82002; 307-777-7531

▪ **Wyoming Health Insurance Pool** (high-risk insurance), 4000 House Avenue, Cheyenne, WY 82003; 800-442-2376 or 307-634-1393

▪ **Wyoming State Health Insurance Information Program**: promotes consumer understanding of Medicare, Medicaid, Medicare supplement, and long-term care insurance. P.O. Box BD, Riverton, WY 82501; 800-856-4398

APPENDIX 2

USEFUL WEB SITES

■ **Agency for Healthcare Research and Quality, www.ahrq.gov.** Provides information in the areas of managed care, mental health, long-term care, and governmental resources.

■ **America's Health Insurance Plans (AHIP), www.ahip.org.** The AHIP is a trade association for companies in the private health care system. The site contains guides on managed care, health insurance, and long-term care and includes an insurance counseling directory.

■ **Center for Medicare and Medicaid Services, www.cms.gov.** Provides information about Medicare, Medicaid, and the State Children's Health Insurance Program (SCHIP).

■ **Center for Medicare Advocacy, www.medicareadvocacy.org.** Nonprofit organization providing legal advice, self-help materials, and representation for elders and people with disabilities who are unfairly denied Medicare coverage.

■ **Dictionary.com, www.dictionary.com.** Online dictionary and thesaurus.

■ **Duke Center for Health Policy, Law and Management, www.hpolicy.duke.edu.** Provides an extensive list of health care links including
  - Federal legislative information on the Thomas web site;
  - Code of federal regulations;
  - Robert Wood Johnson Foundation Web site; and
  - Regional foundations.

■ **Families USA, www.familiesusa.org.** Provides links to documents pertaining to a variety of health care reform issues, including managed care, assistance to the uninsured, and key state bills and legislation.

■ **Free and low-cost prescription drugs**: A listing of drugs whose manufacturers have patient assistance programs:

- www.institute-dc.org

- www.needymeds.com

- www.themedicineprogram.com. Web site for the Medicine Program, an operation that processes applications for patients who cannot afford their prescriptions.

■ **Georgetown University Health Policy Institute, www.healthinsuranceinfo.net.** Comprehensive information describing legal rights and protections regarding health insurance in case studies.

■ **GovSpot, www.govspot.com.** Provides information to online government services including access to public search engines and frequently requested federal 800 numbers.

■ **Health Hippo, http://hippo.findlaw.com.** Hippo is an extensive health information site examining issues ranging from health insurance bills being considered by Congress to the Medicare+Advantage program and the Patient Bill of Rights. Health Hippo also includes an array of search engines providing well over 100 links to other health care sites.

■ **Independent Living Centers, www.ilusa.com/links/ilcenters.htm#AR.** National listing of independent living centers.

■ **Managed Health Care Glossary, www.pohly.com/terms.html.** Provides definitions of terms commonly used by physicians, hospitals, and managed care providers.

■ **Medicare: The Official U.S. Government Site for Medicare Information, www.medicare.gov.** Contains extensive information on Medicare, including access to related websites. Site also provides telephone numbers nationwide to offices familiar with insurers selling Medicare supplement and Medigap coverage, the state's open enrollment policy, and questions pertaining to COBRA, HIPAA, and Medicaid.

The site also provides information on how to apply for drug assistance through drug companies, states, community-based programs, and disease-specific programs. Users can enter their ZIP codes to search for the benefits that are offered in their communities.

Another useful feature is located on the Nursing Home Compare page. Users can obtain and compare information from the Center for Medicare and Medicaid Services' last three surveys of each of the 16,500 nursing homes participating in Medicare and Medicaid. Previously, only the most current survey was available through the site.

- **Medicare Rights Center, www.medicarerights.org.** Offers information to consumers and professionals on Medicare, including counseling by e-mail.

- **National Aging Administration Center, www.aoa.gov,** Site provides extensive information on many issues of interest to the elderly and people with disabilities.

- **National Association of Insurance Commissioners, www.naic.org.** The NAIC is the national organization of state insurance commissioners, and its site concentrates on current state health insurance regulations and policy.

- **National Health Law Program, www.healthlaw.org.** Includes an overview of Medicaid, a fact sheet on the prescription drug programs, and links to state Medicaid sites on the Internet.

- **National Library of Medicine, www.nlm.nih.gov.** Provides access to a number of health organizations, abstracts from over 4,300 biomedical journals, and extensive consumer health information.

- **National Organization of Social Security Claimants' Representatives (NOSSCR), www.nosscr.org.** National organization of attorneys specializing in Social Security matters including Social Security Disability Insurance and Supplemental Security Income. Links to numerous government sites.

- **Pharmaceutical Research and Manufacturers of America (PhRMA), www.phrma.org/patients.** Listing of company programs that provide drugs to physicians whose patients cannot otherwise afford them.

- **Social Security Administration, www.ssa.gov.** Information and forms related to programs of the Social Security Administration, including SSDI and SSI.

- **State and Local Government on the Net, www.statelocalgov.net.** Includes the following for each state:
  - State home page
  - State and local government telephone directory
  - Information pertaining to state's executive, legislative, and judicial branches
  - Information pertaining to county and local offices

- **TRICARE, www.tricare.osd.mil.** An explanation of health benefits available to dependents of veterans.

- **U.S. Department of Labor, www.dol.gov.** Site includes information on the following topics:
  - HIPAA
  - Medicare
  - State Children's Health Insurance Program
  - U.S. Dept. of Health and Human Services consumer health links

- – Federal Employees Health Benefit Plan
- – State insurance departments
- – TRICARE military health system.

■ **Veterans Benefits, www.va.gov.** Site provides information on health benefits available to veterans.

■ APPENDIX 3

DEFINITIONS OF KEY ACRONYMS

COBRA: Consolidated Omnibus Budget Reconciliation Act of 1985

This legislation requires that employers as defined in the act provide employees with continuation of health insurance coverage at group insurance rates when eligibility for employer-related coverage ends. Whether an employee voluntarily resigns or is terminated for any reason other than gross misconduct, those employees protected by COBRA must be given the option of continuing their insurance coverage at their own expense for up to a minimun of 18 months at the group insurance rate. See Chapter 10 for a more detailed explanation.

ERISA: Employee Retirement Income Security Act

ERISA is a federal law that was passed to protect the solvency and security of employee pension plans. However, an unintended benefit of the statute language was to exempt employer health benefit plans from the regulation of state insurance laws if they are self-funded. In self-funded plans, employers set aside revenues to pay the health claims of their workers. Since these benefits are not insurance plans, they are exempt from state insurance laws, including those related to consumer protections. Instead, they are subject to the rules and regulations of the U.S. Department of Labor. Chapter 7 provides a more detailed explanation of ERISA.

HIPAA: Health Insurance Portability and Accountability Act

HIPAA is federal legislation intended to assist individuals when they need to change their group health plan. The law guarantees that most workers who change or lose their jobs will be able to continue to have health insurance without a break in coverage. Eligibility for enrollment in a new group health plan is determined according to the terms of the health plan and the rules of the issuer and not by the insured's health status or any preexisting condition. This protection also applies when transferring to individual health insurance coverage. See Chapter 9 for a more detailed explanation.

SSDI: Social Security Disability Insurance

SSDI is an insurance program for workers unable to work due to long-term disability. It is administered by the Social Security Administration and funded by a tax (referred to as the FICA tax) withheld from the worker's pay and by employer contributions. FICA stands for the Federal Income Contribution Act. See Chapter 4 for a more detailed explanation.

SSI: Supplemental Security Income

SSI is a federal income support program administered by the Social Security Administration. It is a government benefit providing a basic monthly income for individuals who are blind, disabled, or 65 years of age or older and who meet certain financial thresholds. Unlike Social Security Disability Insurance (SSDI), individuals can receive SSI even if they have never worked or would not otherwise qualify for Social Security. See Chapter 5 for a more detailed explanation.

TWWIIA: Ticket to Work and Work Incentives Improvement Act

TWWIIA was enacted in 1999 to make it easier for people with disabilities who are receiving Social Security Disability Insurance to rejoin the workforce without the fear of losing their Medicare or Medicaid coverage. It also provides states with incentives to expand the options and flexibility of their Medicaid programs. See Chapter 12 for a more detailed explanation.

■ APPENDIX 4

STATE PHARMACEUTICAL ASSISTANCE PROGRAMS

Prior to the implementation of the Medicare Modernization Act in 2006, many Medicare beneficiaries lacked coverage for prescription drugs. To help elderly and/or disabled residents access prescription drugs at more affordable prices, many states operated so-called State Pharmaceutical Assistance Programs, or SPAPs. These programs subsidized the cost of prescription drugs for those who were eligible, but varied considerably in their eligibility criteria, benefits, and costs to consumers. They generally required enrollees to pay only a minimal co-pay for their prescriptions.

As prescription coverage under Part D plans in Medicare has become a reality, state legislatures have begun to adapt. Although a few states have eliminated their SPAPs as a result, most have maintained their programs, and a few have even assured that enrollees who are also in a Medicare Part D plan can use the SPAP to "wrap around" or fill in the gaps of their Medicare Part D plan. At this writing, the full implication of the Medicare prescription drug program on SPAPs is still a subject of debate in some state legislatures, and ongoing changes in SPAPs are expected.

The following chart, courtesy of the AARP website, provides an overview of state pharmaceutical programs in place as of December 2004. Because SPAPs are still in the process of change, consumers are strongly encouraged to contact their SPAP or state Department of Aging for up-to-date information about their state's program. The websites of AARP (www.aarp.org). or National Council of State Legislatures (www.ncsl.org) may also have current information about SPAPs.

■ ALABAMA

Alabama SenioRx Partnership for Medication Access

■ **Who qualifies:** Residents age 55 and older with chronic medical conditions who do not have prescription drug coverage

■ **Income restrictions:** Annual income must not exceed $20,000/individual, $26,000/couple

■ **The deal:** SenioRx is a partnership of state agencies and community organizations that assist participants with applying for drug company–sponsored assistance programs.

■ **Cost to join:** None

■ **For details or to apply:** Your local Area Agency on Aging at (800) AGE-LINE (243-5463), or visit the program's website, www.pleasefillin.com.

■ ARIZONA

CoppeRx Card

■ **Who qualifies:** Residents age 65 and older or qualified for Social Security Disability Insurance

■ **Income restrictions:** None

■ **The deal:** Use the card at participating pharmacies when you fill your prescriptions. Discounts typically range from 15 percent to 55 percent off the retail price, depending on medications and pharmacy. While beneficiaries enrolled in Part D can use the card, the cost of prescriptions bought with the card will not count toward one's true out-of-pocket costs to qualify for catastrophic coverage under Medicare Part D.

■ **Cost to join:** None

■ **For details or to apply:** Call RxAmerica at 888-227-8315. Or visit the program's website, www.pleasefillin.com.

■ CALIFORNIA

Prescription Drug Discount Program for Medicare Recipients

■ **Who qualifies:** Medicare beneficiaries without drug coverage

■ **Income restrictions:** None

■ **The deal:** Show your Medicare card at participating pharmacies for varying discounts on prescription drugs. (You'll pay no more than what the Medi-Cal program pays the pharmacy for drugs, plus 15 cents per prescription for a pharmacy administration fee.)

■ **Cost to join:** None

■ **For more details or to apply:** Contact the Department of Health Services at (916) 552-9714 (drug pricing complaints only) or the Health Insurance Counseling and Advocacy Program (HICAP) at (800) 434-0222 (California residents only), or visit the program's website, www.pleasefillin.com.

■ CONNECTICUT

Connecticut Department of Social Services Pharmaceutical Assistance Contract to the Elderly and Disabled (ConnPACE)

■ **Who qualifies:** Low-income residents age 65 and older, or 18 to 64 with a disability

■ **Income restrictions:** Annual income limits of $22,300/individual, $30,100/couple

■ **The deal:** ConnPACE becomes a wrap-around benefit to Part D with extensive coverage for participants, who pay a maximum co-pay of $16.25 per prescription at any point in the Medicare Part D benefit. ConnPACE pays for the monthly drug plan premium for each participant through Dec. 31, 2006, as well as costs prior to, during and after the coverage gap (except for the ConnPACE copay).

■ **Cost to join:** $30 per year

■ **For more details or to apply:** Contact the Department of Social Services at (800) 423-5026 or (860) 832-9265 (local only), or visit the program's website, www.pleasefillin.com.

■ DELAWARE

Delaware Prescription Assistance Program (DPAP)

■ **Who qualifies:** Residents age 65 and older or disabled and qualified for SSDI benefits who don't have prescription drug coverage (excluding Medicare Part D plans)

■ **Income restrictions:** Annual income must not exceed 200 percent of the federal poverty level or have prescription costs that exceed 40 percent of annual income

■ **The deal:** The state's wrap-around program to Part D will cover up to $2,500 of a participant's yearly out-of-pocket costs in certain phases of the Part D benefit: monthly premium toward a basic level prescription drug plan, deductible (a beneficiary must pay either a $5 co-pay or 25 percent of a drug's cost in this phase), and coverage in the gap.

■ **Cost to join:** None

■ **For more details or to apply:** Call the program at (800) 996-9969 (in state only), or visit the program's website, www.pleasefillin.com.

■ FLORIDA

Medicare Prescription Discount Program

■ **Who qualifies:** Medicare beneficiaries

■ **Income restrictions:** None

■ **The deal:** State law lets you show your Medicare card to get a discount based on the average wholesale price minus 9 percent, plus a $4.50 dispensing fee, at pharmacies participating in Florida's Medicaid program. Discounts vary by pharmacy. Program will end in May 2006.

■ **Cost to join:** None

■ **For more details:** Visit your local pharmacist

■ HAWAII

Hawaii Rx Plus Program

■ **Who qualifies:** All state residents

■ **Income restrictions:** Annual income cannot exceed 350 percent of the federal poverty level ($37,464/individual, $50,268/couple)

■ **The deal:** The discount card program lets state residents who do not have prescription drug coverage obtain discounts ranging from 10 percent to 15 percent on medications at participating pharmacies.

■ **Cost to join:** None

■ **For more details:** Oahu residents may call (808) 692-7999 and neighbor island residents may call (866) 878-9769 or visit the program's website, www.pleasefillin.com.

Hawaii State Pharmacy Assistance Program

■ **Who qualifies:** Residents age 65 or older

- **Income restrictions:** Cannot earn more than 100 percent of the federal poverty level ($11,280/individual, $15,180/couple)

- **The deal:** Program will pay for Part D copayments ($1 or $3) of the poorest Hawaiians.

- **Costs to join:** None

- **For more details or to apply:** Oahu residents may call (808) 692-7999 and neighbor island residents may call (866) 878-9769.

■ ILLINOIS

Illinois Cares Rx

- **Who qualifies:** Residents 65 years and older or 16 and older and disabled.

- **Income restrictions:** Participants are eligible in one of two ways: Individuals with income up to $19,140 ($25,660 for couples) are eligible for the Plus set of benefits, while individuals with incomes up to $21,218 ($28,480/couple) qualify for the Basic set of benefits.

- **The deal:** Illinois Cares Rx replaces two drug assistance programs (Illinois SeniorCare and Circuit Breaker) and wraps around Part D coverage by providing assistance with premiums, deductibles, co-pays and costs in the coverage gap. Level of assistance is determined by income. Those qualifying for Plus benefits receive assistance on a wider range of drugs, including some medications excluded from Medicare coverage. Those with slightly higher incomes qualify for Illinois Cares Rx Basic, which assists in the same phases as Plus does, but only for drugs prescribed for Alzheimer's disease, arthritis, cancer, cardiovascular disease, diabetes, glaucoma, Parkinson's disease, lung disease and smoking-related illnesses, multiple sclerosis and osteoporosis.

- **Cost to join or apply:** None

- **For more details or to apply:** Contact the Senior HelpLine at (800) 252-8966, or visit the program's website, www.pleasefillin.com.

Illinois Rx Buying Club

- **Who qualifies:** All uninsured state residents

- **Income restrictions:** Annual income must not exceed 300 percent of the federal poverty level (approximately $60,000 a year for a family of four)

- **The deal:** The discount you get depends on the drug and the pharmacy. You could save up to 24 percent on drug costs, but average savings are 20 percent.

■ **Cost to join:** $10 annual fee
■ **For more details or to apply:** Contact the Buying Club (866)215-3462, or visit the program's website, www.pleasefillin.com.

I-SaveRx

■ **Who qualifies:** Residents of all ages
■ **Income restrictions:** None
■ **The deal:** The program offers residents access to prescription drugs from licensed and inspected pharmacies in Canada, Ireland and the United Kingdom. Discounts vary, but participants can save as much as 80 percent. Drugs purchased through I-SaveRx by Medicare beneficiaries enrolled in Part D will not be credited toward their out-of-pocket drug expenditures.
■ **Cost to join:** None
■ **For more details or to apply:** Call (866) I-SAVE33 (866-472-8333), or visit the program's website, www.pleasefillin.com.

■ INDIANA

HoosieRx

■ **Who qualifies:** Lower-income residents age 65 or older who are enrolled in a Medicare drug plan that works with HoosierRx
■ **Income restrictions:** Must have annual income at or below $14,355 ($19,245/couple)
■ **The deal:** HoosieRx pays the monthly premiums for anyone who isn't receiving full assistance through Medicare and $250 toward any deductible and/or co-pays for participants enrolled in one of four Medicare Part D drug plans working with the program (Community Care Rx BASIC, First Health Premier, PacifiCare Saver Plan or WellCare Signature).
■ **Cost to join:** None
■ **For more details or to apply:** Call (866) 267-4679, or visit the program's website, www.pleasefillin.com.

■ IOWA

Iowa Priority

■ **Who qualifies:** Medicare beneficiaries

- **Income restrictions:** None
- **The deal:** A special discount card program allows beneficiaries until May 31, 2006, to get varying discounts at participating pharmacies on prescriptions.
- **Cost to join:** $20 per year
- **For more details or to apply:** Contact the Iowa Priority Prescription Savings program at (866) 282-5817, or visit the program's website, www.pleasefillin.com.

▪ LOUISIANA

LouisianaSenioRx

- **Who qualifies:** Residents age 60 or older without drug coverage
- **Income restrictions:** Annual income cannot exceed 300 percent of the federal poverty level: $28,710/individual, $38,490/couple
- **The deal:** The program run by the Governor's Office of Elderly Affairs helps qualified residents enroll in prescription assistance programs offered by pharmaceutical companies, helping residents get free or nearly free medicines. The assistance only applies to medications for chronic conditions. No decision has been made on whether the program will continue to help those who enroll in Medicare Part D. If it does, the assistance will only be for medications not covered under Part D.
- **Costs to join:** None
- **For more details or to apply:** Call LouisianaSenioRx at (877) 340-9100, or visit the program's website, www.pleasefillin.com.

▪ MAINE

Maine Rx Plus

- **Who qualifies:** All Maine residents with incomes up to 350 percent of the federal poverty level, or families who spend more than 5 percent of income on prescriptions or 15 percent of income on medical costs
- **Income restrictions:** Monthly income must not exceed $2,793/individual, $3,745/couple
- **The deal:** Show your discount card at participating pharmacies in Maine to save up to 15 percent on brand-name drugs and up to 60 percent on generic drugs.
- **Cost to join:** None

■ **For more details or to apply:** Call (866) RxMaine (796-2463) or (800) 423-4331 (Maine residents only), or visit the program's website, www.pleasefillin.com.

Maine Low Cost Drugs for the Elderly and Disabled Program (DEL)

■ **Who qualifies:** Low-income residents ages 62 and older, or 19 to 61 with a disability

■ **Income restrictions:** Monthly income must not exceed $1,476/individual, $1,980/couple

■ **The deal:** The program expands to become a wrap-around benefit to Medicare Part D for Medicare-eligible individuals with income up to 185 percent of the federal poverty level. The program will provide assistance with copays, deductibles, coverage gap costs and premiums. The amount of assistance is dependent upon individual income and assets.

■ **Cost to join:** None

■ **For more details or to apply:** Contact the Office of Elder Services at (800) 262-2232 or your Local Area Agency on Aging at (877) 353-3771, or visit the program's website, www.pleasefillin.com.

■ MARYLAND

Maryland Senior Prescription Drug Assistance Program

■ **Who qualifies:** Maryland residents eligible for and enrolled in a Medicare prescription drug plan or Medicare Advantage-Prescription Drug (MA-PD) plan

■ **Income restrictions:** Those beneficiaries who have annual income at or below 300 percent of the federal poverty level ($28,710/individual or $38,490/couple) and who do not qualify for federal Extra Help.

■ **The deal:** Participants receive up to $25 per month toward the cost of their monthly Medicare PDP or MA-PD premium.

■ **Cost to join:** None

■ **For more details or to apply:** Contact the Senior Prescription Drug Assistance Program at (800) 551-5995 or (800) 215-8038, or visit the program's website, www.pleasefillin.com.

The Maryland MEDBANK Program

■ **Who qualifies:** Low-income, chronically ill individuals who are uninsured or underinsured. Medbank is unable to assist Medicare patients after Jan. 1, 2006.

- **Income restrictions:** Must have monthly income of at least of $927/individual, $1,074/couple
- **The deal:** This private, nonprofit program helps participants obtain drugs at low or no cost by accessing drug company-run patient assistance programs. Program is designed to help those not qualifying for Maryland assistance programs.
- **Cost to join:** None
- **For more details or to apply:** Call the program at (410) 821-9262 or visit the program's website, www.pleasefillin.com.

■ MASSACHUSETTS

Prescription Advantage

- **Who qualifies:** Residents age 65 and older and certain disabled individuals
- **Income restrictions:** Participants with income up to 500 percent of the federal poverty level ($47,850/individual and $64,150/couple)—but income level determines the amount of assistance a participant receives. Those eligible for full "Extra Help" or who qualify for federal low-income subsidies cannot participate.
- **The deal:** This state insurance program enrolled members in a randomly selected Medicare Part D basic plan and now helps pay for the Medicare Part D premium, deductible and co-payment amounts (including some in the coverage gap). Members may switch plans until May 15, 2006. Now the program is a secondary means of insurance for those with Medicare Part D plans. The amount the program pays is dependent upon income. Meanwhile, traditional coverage still continues for a few thousand program participants who qualify but who don't have Medicare coverage.
- **Cost to join:** None
- **For more details or to apply:** Contact the Office of Elder Affairs at (617) 727-7750. To find help in your area for local service call (800) AGE-INFO (243-4636), or visit the program's website, www.pleasefillin.com.

■ MICHIGAN

MiRx Prescription Savings Program

- **Who qualifies:** All Michigan residents without prescription drug coverage
- **Income restrictions:** Income must be at or below the state's median income, $27,936/individuals, $37,470/couple

■ **The deal:** Show your discount card at participating pharmacies for discounts ranging from 5 percent to 20 percent.

■ **Cost to join:** None

■ **For more details or to apply:** Call (866) 755-6479 or visit the program's website, www.pleasefillin.com.

■ MISSOURI

Missouri Rx Plan (MoRx)

■ **Who qualifies:** Those who are eligible for both Medicare and Medicaid or who were members of the former Missouri Senior Rx Program

■ **Income restrictions:** None aside from those necessary to qualify for Medicare and Medicaid

■ **The deal:** The program wraps around Medicare Part D by paying 50 percent of each individual's out-of-pocket payments, excluding Part D drug plan premium payments.

■ **Cost to join:** None

■ **For more details or to apply:** Contact MoRx at (800) 375-1406, or visit the program's website, www.pleasefillin.com.

■ MONTANA

Big Sky Rx

■ **Who qualifies:** Residents who are enrolled in a Medicare Part D prescription plan

■ **Income restrictions:** Income cannot exceed 200 percent of the federal poverty level ($19,140/individual, $25,660/couple)

■ **The deal:** The program wraps around Medicare Part D for those who do not qualify for full federal assistance by paying up to $33.11 toward the monthly Part D drug plan premium

■ **Costs to join:** None

■ **For more details or to apply:** Call Big Sky Rx at (866) 369-1233 (in state), or (406) 444-1233 (out of state and in the Helena area), or visit the program's website, www.pleasefillin.com.

STATE PHARMACEUTICAL ASSISTANCE PROGRAMS ■ 197

■ NEVADA

Nevada Senior Rx

■ **Who qualifies:** Residents age 62 and older who are not eligible for Medicaid prescription benefits

■ **Income restrictions:** Annual household income must not exceed $23,175/individual, $30,168/couple

■ **The deal:** Those who do not qualify for Medicare are eligible under this cost-sharing program and pay only $10/generic and $25/brand-name drug with an annual coverage limit of $5,100. For Medicare beneficiaries enrolled in a Part D plan, the program will pay up to $23.46 for a participant's monthly Part D plan premium and will pay 100 percent of drug costs for participants during the coverage gap phase.

■ **Cost to join:** None

■ **For more details or to apply:** Contact Senior Rx at (866) 303-6323, or visit the program's website, www.pleasefillin.com.

Nevada Disability Rx

■ **Who qualifies:** Residents ages 18 to 61 with a documented disability who are not eligible for Medicaid prescription benefits

■ **Income restrictions:** Annual household income must not exceed $23,175/individual, $30,168/couple

■ **The deal:** Those who do not qualify for Medicare are eligible under this cost-sharing program and pay only $10/generic and $25/brand-name drug, with an annual coverage limit of $5,100. For Medicare beneficiaries enrolled in a Part D plan, the program will pay up to $23.46 for a participant's monthly Part D plan premium and will pay 100 percent of drug costs for participants during the coverage gap phase.

■ **Cost to join:** None

■ **For more details or to apply:** Contact Senior Rx at (866) 303-6323, or visit the program's website, www.pleasefillin.com.

■ NEW HAMPSHIRE

New Hampshire Medication Bridge Program

■ **Who qualifies:** New Hampshire residents without prescription coverage

■ **Income restrictions:** Monthly household income cannot exceed $1,500/individual, $2,000/couple

■ **The deal:** This privately funded program helps those on medications for chronic conditions secure drugs through pharmaceutical companies. But with several drug companies no longer offering pharmaceutical assistance programs in light of Part D, Medicare-eligible clients may have few options under the Medication Bridge Program.

■ **Cost to join:** None

■ **For more details or to apply:** Call (603) 225-0900, or visit the program's website, www.pleasefillin.com.

■ NEW JERSEY

Pharmaceutical Assistance to the Aged and Disabled (PAAD)

■ **Who qualifies:** Residents age 65 and older or 18 and older and receiving Social Security disability benefits

■ **Income restrictions:** Annual income must not exceed $21,850/individual, $26,791/couple

■ **The deal:** PAAD wraps around Medicare Part D coverage, providing extensive assistance to program participants (who must be enrolled in a Part D PDP and must have applied for a Part D low-income subsidy), who only have to pay a $5 copay for each drug they refill. The program pays premiums, deductibles, co-insurance and other out-of-pocket costs associated with a Medicare Part D drug plan.

■ **Cost to join:** None

■ **For more details or to apply:** Contact the PAAD Hotline at (800) 792-9745, or visit the program's website, www.pleasefillin.com.

Senior Gold Prescription Discount Program

■ **Who qualifies:** Residents age 65 and older or 18 and older and receiving Social Security disability benefits

■ **Income restrictions:** This program serves residents who don't qualify for the state's Pharmaceutical Assistance to the Aged & Disabled program. Annual income must fall within the range of $21,850-$31,850/individual and $26,791-$36,791/couple.

■ **The deal:** Participants enroll and pay the monthly premium for a Medicare Part D program in order for Senior Gold to assist with a beneficiary's other out-of-pocket costs, including deductibles and other co-payments. Senior Gold will also provide some assistance for beneficiaries who choose not to enroll in a PDP, but the state recommends that those with monthly prescription costs of more than $50 enroll in a plan because the savings will likely be greater that way.

■ **Cost to join:** None

■ **For more details or to apply:** Contact the Senior Gold Hotline at (800) 792-9745, or visit the program's website, www.pleasefillin.com.

■ NEW YORK

Elderly Pharmaceutical Insurance Coverage Program (EPIC)

■ **Who qualifies:** Residents of New York State age 65 or older who are not receiving full Medicaid benefits

■ **Income restrictions:** Annual income must not exceed $35,000/single, $50,000/married

■ **The deal:** EPIC is a cost-sharing program covering nearly all prescriptions, including insulin and insulin syringes. Seniors with a maximum yearly income of $20,000/single or $26,000/married pay an annual fee ranging between $8 and $300, depending on income and marital status. Those with higher incomes must pay an annual deductible ranging from $530 to $1,715, depending on income and marital status. After paying the fee or deductible, plan members pay co-pays ranging from $3 to $20, depending on the prescription cost. EPIC will "wrap around" Medicare Part D. Seniors pay a lower co-pay for their medications using Medicare and EPIC together. Except for Part D drug plan premiums, EPIC participants can get Part D deductibles, co-insurance, co-payments, noncovered drugs, or drugs purchased during the coverage gap covered by the state program. Those who qualify for full "Extra Help" and enroll in a Medicare drug plan will have their EPIC enrollment fees waived. They will not pay a premium or deductible for their Medicare drug coverage, and will pay much lower co-payments ($2/generic and $5/brand-name) than with EPIC.

■ **Cost to join:** Annual fee determined by income or deductible referenced above

■ **For more details or to apply:** Call the EPIC Helpline at (800) 332-3742, or access the program's website, www.pleasefillin.com.

■ OHIO

Golden Buckeye Prescription Drug Savings Program

■ **Who qualifies:** Residents age 60 and older, and 18 to 59 with a disability as defined by Social Security

- **Income restrictions:** None
- **The deal:** The program does not work with Medicare Part D, and would be most beneficial to residents who meet program restrictions and who do not have Medicare. Still, it can be applied to prescriptions that are not covered at all by Medicare Part D or another insurance plan. Golden Buckeye cardholders can get discounts averaging 25 percent on a wide range of drugs at most Ohio pharmacies.
- **Costs to join:** None
- **For more details or to apply:** Call the Department of Aging at (866) 301-6446, or visit the program's website, www.pleasefillin.com.

■ OKLAHOMA

Rx for Oklahoma

- **Who qualifies:** Any resident who is uninsured or underinsured
- **Income restrictions:** Up to 300 percent of the federal poverty level typically, but some drug company pharmaceutical assistance programs may have more restricted income guidelines.
- **The deal:** Community action agencies working on behalf of the state's Department of Commerce assist residents in finding and enrolling in pharmaceutical assistance programs sponsored by individual drug companies.
- **Costs to join:** None
- **For more details or to apply:** Call (877) RX4-OKLA (794-6552) (within Oklahoma) or (405) 701-8216.

■ PENNSYLVANIA

Pharmaceutical Assistance Contract for the Elderly (PACE)

- **Who qualifies:** Lower-income residents age 65 and older
- **Income restrictions:** Medicaid qualifiers are not eligible. Annual income limit is $14,500/individual, $17,700/couple
- **The deal:** Currently, members pay co-pays of $6/generic and $9/brand-name prescription. Medicare Part D is changing the way this program works. At this point nothing is certain, but the program's website, www.pleasefillin.com will be updated to reflect changes as they occur.

■ **Cost to join:** None

■ **For more details or to apply:** Contact PACE Cardholder Services at (800) 225-7223 or (717) 651-3600 (outside of Pennsylvania), or visit the program's website, www.pleasefillin.com.

Pharmaceutical Assistance Contract for the Elderly Needs Enhancement Tier (PACENET)

■ **Who qualifies:** Residents age 65 and older who are not eligible for Medicaid

■ **Income restrictions:** Eligible incomes here are slightly higher than for the PACE program. Annual income must not exceed $23,500/individual, $31,500/couple

■ **The deal:** Currently, members pay co-pays of $8/generic and $15/brand-name prescription. Medicare Part D is changing the way this program works. At this point nothing is certain, but the program's website, www.pleasefillin.com will be updated to reflect changes as they occur.

■ **Cost to join:** Participants are subject to a $40 deductible each month

■ **For more details or to apply:** Contact the Pennsylvania Department of Aging at (800) 225-7223 or (717) 651-3600 (outside of Pennsylvania), or visit the program's website, www.pleasefillin.com.

■ RHODE ISLAND

R.I. Pharmaceutical Assistance Program to the Elderly (RIPAE)

For more details or to apply: Contact the Department of Elder Affairs at (401) 462-3000, or visit the program's website, www.pleasefillin.com.

■ SOUTH CAROLINA

Gap Assistance Pharmacy Program for Seniors (GAPS)

■ **Who qualifies:** Medicare beneficiaries enrolled in a Medicare PDP that operates in South Carolina

■ **Income restrictions:** Annual income cannot exceed 200 percent of the federal poverty level

■ **The deal:** Those who qualify pay only 5 percent of the cost of their prescription drugs when they reach Medicare Part D's coverage gap, or "doughnut hole."

■ **Cost to join:** None

■ **For more details or to apply:** Contact the Department of Health and Human Services at (888) 549-0820.

■ TEXAS

Kidney Health Care Program

■ **Who qualifies:** Residents with end-stage renal disease or kidney transplant patients

■ **Income restrictions:** Income cannot exceed $60,000 annually

■ **The deal:** Medicare beneficiaries eligible for the program get their Part D premiums (Basic plan only, up to $35) paid for and their co-pay first four renal-related prescriptions on their Part D plan's formulary. Travel benefits and other costs involved with dialysis are also included. For program participants without Medicare coverage, the program pays for the full cost of the first four renal-related prescriptions.

■ **Costs to join:** None

■ **For more details or to apply:** Call the program at (800) 222-3986 or (512) 458-7150 (in Austin), or visit the program's website, www.pleasefillin.com.

■ VERMONT

Vermont Pharmacy Program (VPharm)

■ **Who qualifies:** Medicare recipients

■ **Income restrictions:** Program offers three tiers of eligibility with the upper-income limit running to 225 percent of the federal poverty level. Monthly income must not exceed $1,795/individual, $2,406/couple.

■ **The deal:** The state's VHAP and VSCRIPT programs have become VPharm, a pharmacy assistance program with three levels of benefits determined by income. Tier 1: Those with incomes up to 150 percent of the federal poverty level ($1,197/individual, $1,604/couple per month) pay $13 a month and get coverage for acute and maintenance drugs and all Part D drug plan premiums (up to $30.27 a month), deductibles, co-pays and co-insurance obligations. Part D-excluded drugs are covered to the extent that they would have been covered by VHAP prior to Part D and VPharm. Tier 2: Those with incomes up to 175 percent of the federal poverty level ($1,396/individual, $1,872/couple per month) pay $17 a month in order to get coverage of the Part D premium and cost-sharing for maintenance drugs. Tier 3: Those earning up to 225 percent of the federal poverty level (see above for monthly income limits) pay $35 a month in order to get the same benefits as those eligible for Tier 2. Coverage of Part D-excluded drugs is limited to drugs for which the manufacturer has signed a state-only rebate agreement. All three tiers receive coverage in the "doughnut hole" as defined by their program.

- **Cost to join:** Monthly premiums as described above
- **For more details or to apply:** Contact the Office of Vermont Health Access at (800) 250-8427, or visit the program's website, www.pleasefillin.com.

Healthy Vermonters Discount Program

- **Who qualifies:** All state residents with incomes below 300 percent of the federal poverty level, Medicare beneficiaries with incomes below 400 percent of the federal poverty level.
- **Income restrictions:** Medicare beneficiaries' monthly income must not exceed $2,994/individual, $4004/couple. Other qualifiers' monthly income must not exceed $2,245/individual, $3,300/couple
- **The deal:** Cardholders get to purchase drugs at the rate the state Medicaid program pays. Medicare beneficiaries who qualify will be able to purchase only those drugs that Part D does not cover by law, including drugs for anorexia, weight loss, weight gain, smoking cessation, over-the-counter prescriptions, barbiturates and benzodiazepines.
- **Cost to join:** No cost
- **For more details or to apply:** Call at (800) 250-8427, or visit the program's website, www.pleasefillin.com.

■ WASHINGTON

Rx Washington

- **Who qualifies:** All state residents
- **Income restrictions:** No income restrictions on the revamped program

■ **The deal:** The card allows individuals 5 percent to 25 percent discounts on drugs through either mail order or retail pharmacies in the Express Scripts national network of pharmacies.

■ **Cost:** $10 per year

■ **For more details or to apply:** Call (800) 227-5255 or visit the program's website, www.pleasefillin.com.

■ WEST VIRGINIA

Golden Mountaineer Discount Card

■ **Who qualifies:** Residents age 60 and older

■ **Income restrictions:** None

■ **The deal:** A special discount card program, not a Part D wrap-around, gives cardholders varying discounts at participating stores on all prescription drugs as well as some retail products and professional services. The state says Medicare beneficiaries can use it in certain circumstances, such as buying drugs in the coverage gap. It cannot be used for co-pays charged by a prescription plan.

■ **Cost to join:** None **For more details or to apply:** Contact the Bureau of Senior Services at (304) 558-3317 or toll-free at (877) 987-3646, or visit the program's website, www.pleasefillin.com.

■ WISCONSIN

SeniorCare

■ **Who qualifies:** Residents age 65 and older who are not eligible for Medicaid

■ **Income restrictions:** The program has four levels of benefits. Level 1: maximum yearly income of $15,680/individual, $21,120/couple. Level 2A: maximum yearly income of $19,600/individual, $26,400/couple. Level 2B: maximum yearly income of $23,520/individual or $31,680/couple. Level 3: yearly income over $23,521/individual or $31,681/couple

■ **The deal:** Senior Care is considered creditable coverage for Medicare Part D. Participants have a choice of staying in the program and paying only $5 per generic or $15 per brand-name drug. Most drugs are covered, with co-pays and deductibles determined by the assigned benefit level.

■ **Cost to join:** $30 enrollment fee per person

■ **For more details or to apply:** Call the program toll-free at (800) 657-2038, or visit the program's website, www.pleasefillin.com.

■ WYOMING

Prescription Drug Assistance Program

■ **Who qualifies:** All state residents who do not have prescription drug coverage

■ **Income restrictions:** Income must not exceed 100 percent of the federal poverty level ($9,570/individual, $12,830/couple)

■ **The deal:** Purchase up to three drugs a month for a $10 co-pay per generic or $25 copay per brand-name prescription at participating pharmacies.

■ **Cost to join:** None

■ **For more details or to apply:** Contact the Department of Family Services at (307) 777-7921 or the Department of Health at (800) 438-5785, or visit the program's website, www.pleasefillin.com.

Reprinted from the April 2006 issue of AARP Bulletin Online, a publication of AARP. Compiled by Christopher J. Gearon. Copyright 2006 AARP. All rights reserved.

■ APPENDIX 5

STATE CHILDREN'S HEALTH INSURANCE PROGRAM

In 1997 Congress adopted legislation to assist states in providing health insurance coverage to children from working families with incomes too high to qualify for Medicaid but too low for them to afford private insurance. Titled the State Children's Health Insurance Program, or SCHIP, each state with an approved plan receives federal matching funds for its plan's expenditures. As early as 2002, all 50 states, the District of Columbia, and five U.S. territories had programs approved by the federal Department of Health and Human Services.

The legislation sets eligibility criteria while providing each state discretionary authority to narrow the standard for those children targeted to be covered under its program. Premiums charged by a state must be based on an income-related sliding scale. There can be a variety of immigration statuses within the family.

In most states, children under the age of 19 are eligible for SCHIP coverage if their families earn less than $36,100 per year for a family of four (2006). Although benefits vary from state to state, most states cover

- ■ Doctor visits
- ■ Immunizations
- ■ Hospitalizations
- ■ Emergency room visits

Almost 4 million children are covered under the SCHIP program. However, the dramatic decrease in state revenues experienced over recent years has made it difficult for states to maintain or increase funding for this program and continue the outreach and enrollment simplification needed to find and enroll eligible families.

At the same time, continued erosion of employer health coverage, especially among employers offering low-wage jobs, makes SCHIP an important source of health coverage for many families that rely on these jobs. There is no question that federal decisions on reauthorization of SCHIP funding, and the reallocation of funding to states that exceed their allotment, will be critical to future state decisions regarding SCHIP coverage.

A status report and contact information regarding State Children's Health Insurance Programs can be obtained from the website of the Center for Medicare and Medicaid Services (www.cms.gov). One can also telephone for information at 877-KIDS-NOW (877-543-7669).

Index